Making Tough
Decisions about
End-of-Life Care
in Dementia

A 36-Hour Day Book

# Making Tough Decisions about End-of-Life Care in Dementia

**Anne Kenny, MD**

Johns Hopkins University Press
Baltimore

This book is not meant to substitute for medical, legal, or other professional care of people with dementia, and treatment should not be based solely on its contents. Instead, treatment must be developed in a dialogue between the individual and his or her physician. This book has been written to help with that dialogue.

© 2018 Anne Kenny
All rights reserved. Published 2018
Printed in the United States of America on acid-free paper
9 8 7 6 5 4 3 2 1

Johns Hopkins University Press
2715 North Charles Street
Baltimore, Maryland 21218-4363
www.press.jhu.edu

Library of Congress Cataloging-in-Publication Data

Names: Kenny, Anne, 1959– author.
Title: Making tough decisions about end-of-life care in dementia / Anne Kenny.
Description: Baltimore : Johns Hopkins University Press, 2018. | Series:
    A 36-hour day book | Includes bibliographical references and index.
Identifiers: LCCN 2018004456| ISBN 9781421426662 (hardcover : alk. paper) |
    ISBN 1421426668 (hardcover : alk. paper) | ISBN 9781421426679 (paperback :
    alk. paper) | ISBN 1421426676 (paperback : alk. paper) | ISBN 9781421426686
    (electronic) | ISBN 1421426684 (electronic)
Subjects: | MESH: Terminal Care—standards | Dementia | Caregivers—
    psychology | Decision Making | Suicide, Assisted | Aged | Personal Narratives
Classification: LCC RC521 | NLM WM 220 | DDC 616.8/31029—dc23
LC record available at https://lccn.loc.gov/2018004456

A catalog record for this book is available from the British Library.

*Special discounts are available for bulk purchases of this book. For more information, please contact Special Sales at 410-516-6936 or specialsales@press.jhu.edu.*

Johns Hopkins University Press uses environmentally friendly book materials, including recycled text paper that is composed of at least 30 percent post-consumer waste, whenever possible.

*To Mom who taught us so much as she lived well
and died from dementia*

# Contents

# Preface

This book is laid out as a guidebook. Nearly 500,000 individuals are diagnosed with dementia every year. Year after year. As stunning as that figure is, it does not take into account the family members and caregivers who are subsequently affected by each diagnosis. When they are included, the numbers rise to an even more incredible level.

What this means in our society is a rapidly ballooning population of people faced with painful scenarios and the need to make vital end-of-life decisions for those who no longer can—a role for which most are largely unprepared. Sadness, confusion, guilt, anger, and physical and mental exhaustion become the norm for these families as the disease enters its final stage. The toughest decisions I ever made were about the life and death of my mother, who had lost her voice in decisions to dementia. But, I was one of the lucky ones. My 25 years as a doctor specializing in the care of older people and end-of-life care had prepared me to face these decisions. Yet, even with that advantage, I struggled. The challenges that dementia and end-of-life decisions present usually are overwhelming. My personal experience compelled me to fuse my clinical knowledge with everything I learned helping to care for my mother into a book to help others.

This book is a guide focused on *care* and *decision*s in the final stages of dementia. Specifically, it is meant to help you deal with inevitable end-of-life problems, such as pain and difficulties with eating, and show you how to navigate the difficult decision-making challenges and communication needs among caregivers and health care providers in the final stages.

The guide may be read as a whole, to give you a landscape for what types of decisions and issues surrounding care and communication may arise along the journey with dementia. Also, if you have questions about care issues specific to the end stage of dementia, you can review the relevant chapter. For example, many families want to know more about what happens in the final weeks or days of life to prepare themselves or other family members—this can be found in chapter 7.

Each chapter includes stories of families I've met and worked with during the past 30 years. These stories are meant to illustrate a common issue, concern, or situation that occurs in late-stage dementia. I hope that by seeing how others have met these challenges, you will see a way to go forward also.

The names of all the people involved have been changed. Identifying characteristics such as ages, genders, ethnicities, professions, familial relationships, medical situations, and social situations have been changed to protect the identities of those involved. At times, a composite of a few people or families was created to illustrate a point. Any resemblance to persons living or dead resulting from these changes is coincidental and unintentional.

# Acknowledgments

There are so many people to thank for making this book possible. I am grateful for all I've learned from all of them in the process of writing it.

First, I would like to thank my mother, my siblings (Hugh, Marilyn, Crazy Dog, Mary Fran, Jack, Donna, Joe, and Connie), and their children and my immediate family (Mark, Conor, Ned, and Becky) for making our personal journey with Alzheimer disease enlightening, rewarding, and rich. The joy and sorrow of living the journey with you transformed my life. My mother had an amazing spirit and passed it down to her children—we are lucky. My immediate family was always there with a meal, a hug, patience, laughs, companionship, and love to me and my mother during the years preceding her death. There are no words to thank you all.

Next, this book would not be possible without the generous patients and families that allowed me to enter their lives, to witness their adaptability in the face of a relentless disease. I've been changed by knowing all of you and am grateful.

I would like to thank Jacqueline Wehmueller, a former acquisitions editor for Johns Hopkins University Press, who first encouraged the kernel of an idea; that encouragement was vital to taking the first step. And then further thanks to Susan Aiello, DVM, who helped to water and prune the plant until there was a completed book; she was always ready with a kind word, a gentle nudge, cheer, and a strong rewrite. Julie Silver, MD, hosted an amazing writing conference that provided the framework to move the idea to a book. Martha Murphy provided early coaching to develop a book proposal.

Thank you to the University of Connecticut "SISters" writing group (Julie, Noreen, Liisa, and Lisa) for weekly accountability and encouragement. A particular thanks to Noreen for assistance and resources that made a physician writing on legal aspects of end of life less daunting. Thanks also to Barbara and Terran at Farmington River Financial Group for assistance and guidance in drafting the financial aspects of the book. The "PalGals" (Cassandra, Katy, and Patty) taught me so much about caring and compassion at the end of life. Theresa kept me sane and mindful. Denise, Pam, Annmarie, Chris, Kelly, and Catherine provided just the right amount of cheerleading to keep me going. Finally, love and thanks to ALK for reading, clarification, suggestions, daily walks, drying tears, and continuous encouragement, love, and support—I couldn't have done it without you.

Making Tough
Decisions about
End-of-Life Care
in Dementia

# Introduction

---

## BEGINNING THE PROCESS OF LETTING GO

### • *The Kenny Family Story* •

The time had come. I had seen it coming. My sister called to let me know my mother had been admitted to the hospital for the second time in 10 days. The call signaled the change in my mother I had been both waiting for and dreading. Once a vibrant, laughing life of the party, my mother had become quiet, tentative, almost shy. She had always been known for her laughing eyes, her love of song and dance, and her playful spirit. When one of her six children needed discipline, with a twinkle in her eye, she would threaten to hit us with a board, quickly upping the ante to a board with a nail, followed by a board with a rusty nail if we kept up our antics. We never met the end of that board, with or without the nail, although she had our attention as she reprimanded us with love and tenderness. But now, she was distant and reserved. Her usual sparkle was lost, replaced by a look of fright or uncertainty. She had our attention again.

The changes signaled the late stages of her 10-year journey with dementia. She lay in the hospital bed, ignoring her limp right side. A lopsided smile, when she could muster one on her mostly sad face, was too often punctuated by flashes of anger as she attempted to make herself understood but could not come up with any words or, worse yet, the wrong ones. These changes had been brought on by a stroke that took even more of her memory, personality, speech, and strength. In the last year or so, my mother had begun the process of *letting go*. She was letting go of her loves—travel, her home, her husband, her independence, her twinkling eyes.

---

1

## CONVERSATIONS ABOUT DEATH AND LETTING GO

As a geriatrician and palliative care physician with more than 25 years of experience, my goal is to help families give a voice to the person whose voice has been lost to late-stage dementia. Luckily, some have had the conversation about how they would like to live through to the end of their disease during the early stages when their voices were strong and clear, making letting go easier for their families. But many others avoid the conversation, because discussing death and the process of dying is uncomfortable and, to some, taboo. Even those who waded into the waters of discussion of facing death likely did not reach the level of detail needed by families as they grapple with the day-to-day decisions when dementia has progressed to the late stages—decisions about when to feed or not, when to give antibiotics or not, when to stay at home rather than being transferred to the hospital. Making decisions yet even more difficult is the possibility of "push back" from health care providers, who reflexively maintain life and are often most uncomfortable addressing death. Finally, it does not help anyone facing these choices that dementia is accompanied by a variable and unpredictable decline.

Persons living with cancer, who usually maintain their voice, are pioneers in training health care providers in the possibility of honoring a less medicalized version of the end of life. There are lessons to learn from death—the ability to see death as a liberation and a time for growth, rather than resisting its inevitability with tubes, wires, and machines. The time has come to offer the same holistic approach to those living and dying with Alzheimer disease and related dementias.

---

### RESISTING THE PROGRESSION OF DISEASE
#### • Theresa's Story •

Theresa's small, cherub's face, along with her white hair and smooth skin, hid her chronological age. She was in her early 90s and, for the first time since I met her, sat with her shoulders slumped. She had buried her lifelong love, Herb, three months earlier. Herb had lived with dementia for eight years—six years active and engaged, two years in bed and withdrawn. I had shared in Herb's care for about six-and-a-half years, but then Theresa and Herb's children requested to continue Herb's care with another physician. They felt that Herb's decrease in activity and mobility, along with his weight loss, should be aggressively challenged. Theresa was caught between what I described as the progression of dementia and the desire to follow the advice of her children (and the hope that they were right and that Herb would "perk up" with physical therapy, aggressive nutrition, and stimulation).

Theresa was reliving with me Herb's course since I had last seen him 18 months earlier. She described exhaustion from transferring Herb into and out of a wheelchair to get him to physical therapy three times per week, from cooking six meals per day, from constantly coaxing him to eat a few bites. Herb would often have angry outbursts when she woke him to eat, move, or talk. She poked and prodded him to "lure him back to life." After about a year, she heard a small voice telling her she was not helping either Herb or herself. As she began to relax, Herb rested and she did, too. But then her children started up. "Why isn't he eating?" "He's losing too much weight!" "He can't even help us when we try to walk him to the bathroom anymore." The children took turns living with Herb and Theresa to help with the eating, exercise, and stimulation. When Herb died in the hospital from complications of a urinary tract infection, Theresa said the entire family was exhausted and angry, questioning what else they could have done. There was no peace or acceptance of death.

---

## DEMENTIA IS A CHRONIC BUT *TERMINAL* DISEASE, NO MATTER HOW MUCH CARE WE GIVE

Is there another way? I spoke with a new friend who had spent 11 years caring for her husband. She now works to assist others in coping with care partnering, because she doesn't want others to have to learn by trial and error what she had to learn and come to accept on her own during her time as a care partner. She said that, even with all she learned, she thought she could keep her husband from dying. She felt her care partnering and caregiving would protect him from death and from leaving her. She says she finds this sentiment to be true in many of her caregiving support groups. She now tries to ease the groups into understanding that there is a time that we will die . . . even from dementia.

Dementia, the sixth leading cause of death in the United States, has different stages: the early and mid-stages in which individuals continue to participate in many of their typical activities, and the late stages with the hallmarks of severe disability. The typical features of advanced dementia are profound memory deficits, limited verbal abilities, impaired ability to walk independently, and loss of the ability to perform activities of daily living (for example, bathing, dressing, and toileting). At this stage of dementia, life expectancy is typically only a little more than a year. Most individuals have difficulty eating, their swallowing muscles forgetting the steps to chew, swallow, and protect their breathing tube. The result is pneumonia, often repeated bouts, from aspiration. In studies done by investigators at Harvard Medical School, 90 percent of those making decisions for individuals with advanced dementia state their goal is for comfort, moving away from goals for treatment or cure. Yet, approximately 16 percent of those who die with dementia do so in the hospital, and reports show that 20 percent of those with dementia have multiple transitions or hospitalizations in the last 90 days of life.

---

### SHIFTING FOCUS FROM CURE TO COMFORT
#### • Mary and Ted's Story •

When I first spoke with Mary, a petite woman with warm, deep brown eyes, she never took her hand off Ted. Ted was long, lean, and asleep but with the droopy, drooling face that accompanies oversedation. Ted's wrists were restrained and an intravenous line snaked into his left arm, an arm wrapped above and below the elbow onto a thin, padded board designed to keep his arm from bending and kinking the intravenous tubing. The sheets had been kicked off his legs, and I could see a catheter in place so that Ted did not urinate into the bed. Mary looked embarrassed as I quickly scanned the room and the situation. "I'm afraid to move the sheets or speak too loudly for fear of waking him and having him yank at all his tubes. He just finally settled down. He gets so angry and afraid. He just thrashes around—the thrashing scares me. It's bad enough at home when he gets upset, but here he is connected to all these wires and gizmos. I know he would be appalled at being in the bed without being covered." Her eyes well with tears. "I just never know whether to bring him here for this . . ." She motions at the intravenous bag, the hospital room, and Ted tied to the bed. "Or what would happen if we just stayed home?"

After Mary spoke a little longer about her and Ted's 45 years of marriage, their children, and their life, I began to bring the conversation back to Ted. His diagnosis, his stage of dementia, the reasons for bringing him into the hospital over the last year, and her initial query: what would happen if they just stayed home? Ted had reached the final stage of dementia. He was sleeping 14 to 16 hours a day and had lost his ability to speak. Mary described only short periods of "meaningful interaction." Whenever Ted's behavior changed—he would become more aggressive or sometimes sedate—Mary knew health care providers would find a urinary tract infection or pneumonia. I discussed with Mary the usual course for dementia in the late stages. "It is a relief to hear from someone that this is the typical situation. No one has ever talked about what happens as the disease gets worse. I always think I haven't taken good enough care of Ted and that is why he is declining." We discussed what would happen if they stayed home the next time he was sick. "But, how can I not treat something that is fixable?" It is the question I'm asked most often and the reason for this book.

## HOW WE SEE DEATH AND HOW OUR
## VISIONS ARE CHANGING

National conversations about dying are beginning. In *Being Mortal*, Dr. Atul Gawande, a surgeon at the Brigham and Women's Hospital in Boston, Massachusetts, and frequent contributor to the *New Yorker*, explores our national and cultural medicalized dealings with aging, frailty, and death. Dr. Gawande posits that we may want to bring meaning and well-being back to the forefront, rather than survival and safety. I now have people talking with me at parties and barbecues about the concept of "allowing death"—conversations that did not happen 10 years ago.

Michael Hebb, described as an innovative and influential cultural figure, entrepreneur, and activist who uses food and the dinner table to provoke discussions and connections, began the "Let's have dinner and talk about death" movement—an idea that came to him as he was commuting on a train, discussing the state of health care in the United States with two other travelers, both physicians. He learned on that trip that although 75 percent of individuals would like to die at home, only 25 percent do. He also learned that a staggering majority of bankruptcies are due to end-of-life health care costs. He personally admits that one of his only regrets is not spending more time with his father during his final years living with and dying from Alzheimer dementia.

In April 2016, Hebb estimated that about 10,000 "Death over Dinner" events had occurred in 30 countries. The website http://deathoverdinner.org/ describes how to host an event, with supporting materials to choose from to personalize how to enhance reflection, introspection, and conversation. Those involved in these dinners find that speaking of death can be moving, cathartic, warm, and liberating. You may find that having the courage to start such a discussion, with prompts suggested by Hebb, including good food (and maybe libations), will lead to some interesting and surprising insights and revelations.

Other movements such as 5 Wishes, Compassion and Choices, and the Conversation Project move discussions forward to understand

and deliberate advance directives and articulate choices and wishes for the end of life. Physicians and other health care workers are not currently trained to think about letting go—but this is changing. The John A. Hartford Foundation, an organization dedicated to improving the care of older adults, released information that only 29 percent of primary care physicians received training in end-of-life discussions, although nearly all believed that this type of physician-patient discussion should occur. The introduction of Vital Talks, a program geared to health care providers to aid in the "how" to have difficult conversations in palliative care, is spurring spin-offs specific to oncology, emergency medicine, and other specialties.

All these efforts by the health care community are a good beginning, but they may not reach your neighborhood in time for you and your family. In the hospital where I work, I know I will be in a meeting with family members, hospitalists, and other specialists, and no one will be directly talking about the process of dying. When it is finally brought up, the entire room seems somehow to physically relax. Shoulders lower and faces soften, and we can begin the real conversation that we know we are there for. The conversation may have sad elements, but the need for the conversation is real and the situation is often better dealt with directly.

---

## RECOGNIZING THAT DIRECTION MAY NOT COME FROM THE HEALTH CARE COMMUNITY
### • Dr. Key •

I was approached by the nursing supervisor, Tessa, from the medical floor, asking if she could speak to me in a small conference room. She pulled up a chair and sighed and then leaned in close and said, "Can you please talk with Dr. Key? We all know she hates to see someone die, but this is getting ridiculous. The family wants to take Mr. Jacques in Room 23 home to die, but she is pressuring them to get a feeding tube, at least for a three-month trial." Tessa described Mr. Jacques as being in the late stages of dementia. He'd been admitted every month for the last six months with a range of maladies, including urinary tract infection, influenza, and dehydration. He was losing weight, awake for only a few hours every day, and in no need of medications. His children had all come together to assure Mrs. Jacques that further medical treatment was not necessary to keep Dad alive; they wanted to support their mother in whatever decision she felt was right for her husband. Once Mrs. Jacques knew her children supported her, she admitted she felt the last year or so had been torture for her husband, and it was time to stay home and keep him comfortable. No more back and forth to the hospital.

Dr. Key was asked to come to a family meeting to hear this decision, but she told the family that because most of his admissions were for dehydration, he could be kept hydrated at home with a feeding tube. The family reacted with anger and confusion and asked Dr. Key to leave so they could discuss the new information among themselves. Mrs. Jacques held her face in her hands and cried. She did not want to give up on her husband if there was a chance for improved quality of life, but the mixed messages from the medical community confused her.

I approached Dr. Key and asked what her understanding was of Mr. Jacques' condition, prognosis, and goals of care. Her eyes flashed angrily and then quickly looked away. "He just can't keep up his hydration. A feeding tube seems the best course of action." I asked for what outcome was it the best course? "So he can *live*." She emphasized the last word very heavily. I sat quietly for a minute waiting to see if she had anything else to say. Dr. Key began to cry, softly and quietly. She whispered, "It just gets so hard to see all these people die. I just want to do something to help them." I continued to wait. "I can't just offer nothing." I asked, "Is that what you think? That you have nothing to offer?" Dr. Key nodded and asked, "Don't you?" I said there is so much to offer—compassion, an ear, an opinion, and understanding. Dr. Key said, "It doesn't seem enough."

---

# HEALTH CARE PROVIDERS ARE TRAINED
# TO PREVENT MORTALITY

Dr. Gawande, in *Being Mortal*, describes the medical profession as one that sees a problem and then fixes it, but with aging, frailty, and dementia, there are no real fixes, thus leading to suffering rather than comfort. "This experiment of making mortality a medical experience is just decades old. It is young. And the evidence is it is failing. . . . Our reluctance to honestly examine the experience of aging and dying has increased the harm we inflict on people and denied them the basic comforts they most need (p. 9)."

My goal in this book is to assist families in understanding the current focus of society and health care on preventing mortality. From this understanding, families will be better able to advocate with health care professionals to obtain the best care for a family member who is in the end stages of dementia. The conversation, led by those with the needs of their family at the center, will expand to include other decision makers, family members, physicians, long-term care administrators, and staff for day-to-day decisions. In time, the conversation needs to extend to legislators and cultural leaders who articulate the thoughts of the country. A palliative approach to care at the end of life for those living with dementia means shifting our perspective to focus on goals of connection and comfort and away from procedures, hospitals, and life at all costs.

——————— **POINTS TO REMEMBER** ———————

▶ Discussions regarding death from dementia are not happening among family members, health care workers, and the community.

▶ The lack of understanding and discussion about signs and symptoms that signal late-stage dementia may contribute to the lack of conversations regarding wishes for end-of-life care in family members with dementia.

▸ Those living with late-stage dementia often are subjected to multiple hospitalizations and medical procedures when reports suggest those who make decisions for them, or surrogate decision makers, favor comfort.

▸ A national dialogue on accepting death into the medical model of disease is taking root, so that more families and health care providers are making decisions that focus on connection and comfort rather than on prolonging survival at the end of life, such as during late-stage dementia.

## ACTION PLAN

▸ Be brave enough to begin conversations about death and about you and your family's wishes for how to die using one of several platforms described in the text, such as Death over Dinner or the Conversation Project.

▸ Educate yourself about the signs and symptoms of the last stage of dementia so you are ready to deliberate the right course of action based on the prognosis in late stages.

▸ If your family chooses comfort rather than a curative approach, seek out the assistance of a palliative care team that focuses on a holistic approach to navigate the health care system for your family member.

## ADDITIONAL READING AND RESOURCES

▸ *Embracing Our Mortality: Hard Choices in an Age of Medical Miracles*, by Lawrence J. Schneiderman

Written by a physician with many years of experience as a medical ethicist, this book reviews some of the current issues facing individuals receiving health care in the United States. Dr. Schneiderman makes the case for embracing our mortality and educates us on how well medical decisions are made by individuals and those who care for them. The book is not specific to those with dementia but clearly articulates ethical terms and conditions so that all sides of a complex medical situation can be evaluated.

▶ *Hard Choices for Loving People: CPR, Feeding Tubes, Palliative Care, Comfort Measures, and the Patient with a Serious Illness,* 6th ed., by Hank Dunn

This short guide, written by an ordained health care chaplain, covers common medical decisions encountered at the end of life. He provides brief statistics on how often procedures are chosen and what the outcomes are. He also provides different ways to emotionally or spiritually approach these decisions.

# Understanding the End and the Need for Letting Go

If you are reading this book, you realize that your family member is moving to the final stages of dementia. More than 5 million Americans are living with dementia, a progressive brain disease that, as it marches to its final stages, means affected individuals will require more and more assistance from caregivers. But how do we know those final stages are nearing? And what does it mean for caregivers, not just physically but emotionally as well?

---

### RECOGNIZING THE END IS NEARING
#### • *The Kenny Family Story* •

My mom gave birth to six independently minded children, all with big personalities—a nice way of saying we do well when things go the way we see it, but struggle when they don't. Understanding that my mom's dementia had moved to the end stages came to my siblings and me at different times. My mom often didn't wake until 11 a.m., rubbing the sleep from her eyes, but quickly responded to coaxing and miming to put her arm out so we could put on her sweater, humming along with me as I readied her toothbrush.

On a day like this, some of the Kenny kids would interpret Mom as doing great. Others realized that for this one hour of calm and cooperative dressing, she needed 12 hours of sleep. We recognized the probability that within an hour or two, Mom would offer only a blank stare. When she was able to focus, we recognized the mom from our youth and worried we were approaching her care from too negative a lens or missing some need that would unlock the path to full recovery. But gradually, one by one, we all saw that Mom barely spoke, coughed on a sip of juice, walked with less and less assuredness, and needed more and more sleep.

---

As dementia progresses to final stages, affected individuals will require more and more assistance from caregivers. The staggering majority of caregivers are family and loved ones. Information on caregivers reveals several interesting facts: Most live with the family member receiving care, with more than half providing more than 20 hours of care per week. Two-thirds of caregivers are younger than retirement age, suggesting they either work outside the home, care for small children, or both. The price of caregiving is high, both financially and emotionally, but so are the benefits. The burdens and benefits escalate as the disease progresses. Caregivers clearly appreciate the need to be available to provide help, but the intensity and persistence of that care is daunting.

I loved being able to care for my mom. In fact, I felt honored. When coworkers offered sympathy for having to take time to care for her, I honestly reported I felt privileged to care for and continue to learn from her. But, at the same time, I felt crushed by the responsibility and what appeared like a long road ahead. I felt both gratitude and troubled at the same time, a mix of emotions similar to that reported by many patients' family members.

---

## RECOGNIZING AND ADAPTING
## TO PROGRESSION OF DEMENTIA
### • *Kathleen and Dottie's Story* •

For many years, Kathleen, an acquaintance from work, often pulled me aside to tell me about her mother, Dottie. At first, Kathleen reported extreme frustration with her mother's stubbornness. Dottie, usually outgoing and "spunky," would no longer drive to her brother's house for a holiday party; she now "expected her children to cater to her." Usually so confident and self-assured, Dottie had started to become anxious and worry about silly things like weather reports and if "the grandkids were all right." Once we discovered that Dottie was suffering from memory loss, Kathleen's compassion for her mother grew as she realized these irritating new habits or demands likely stemmed from Dottie's memory loss and her efforts to adapt to it. Kathleen found joy in working with her mother to decrease Dottie's anxiety and allow her continued independence.

As Dottie's dementia progressed, Kathleen would pull me aside, again with frustration at her mother's new state. Finally, one day as Kathleen rushed toward me with a knitted brow, we both started laughing. "I must be looking for a new way of coping with the next stage, right?" she asked. I nodded. Over coffee, we discussed what was *not* working and began brainstorming strategies that Kathleen could take back to her mother and family for the trial and error required to find a new path forward. Dottie eventually moved into a skilled nursing facility as her care needs escalated to requiring assistance with daily bathing and toileting, care she was uncomfortable accepting from her children. Although the children first argued about who should be providing care, after they observed their mother accepting care from others who were not family members, they understood that this was the best choice for Dottie.

## THE TRANSITION TO END-STAGE DISEASE

### Overview of the Functional Stages of Dementia

Dementia is a cluster of neurodegenerative diseases that impair several aspects of functioning, including memory, language, ability to complete complex tasks, social skills, judgment and reasoning, and several motor functions such as walking and swallowing. In this overview, the focus will be on Alzheimer dementia—the most common form of dementia—and issues that occur in the later stages of dementia. You've likely already seen several issues in your family member in the earlier stages, such as personality changes; behaviors that may not have made sense such as paranoia, hoarding, or wandering; loss of the ability to use the correct word and the subsequent frustration in expression; loss of the ability to safely drive; or the beginning of a shuffling walking style.

While there are several ways to understand the progression of dementia, I have found that focusing on function assists in planning for changes in care needs, housing, approach, and adaptation. How do we know when someone has moved to the end stages of dementia? In cancer, for example, disease has progressed when atypical cells are found in lymph nodes or have spread to bone. But in dementia, each case is different. There is no clear classification when the disease has officially crossed the line from mild to moderate to severe. There is no "typical" course. Even so, function, defined as the ability to get things done, may be used as a common thread and guidepost that can assist caregivers in care and decision making.

The Functional Assessment Staging Tool (FAST)* scale is a commonly used measure to guide health care professionals in staging dementia for prognosis and resource recommendation. It is based on functional ability more than other measures. Table 1.1 outlines the FAST scale with the stage of dementia and the commonly associated clinical patterns. In moderate and severe stages of dementia, the scale becomes more specific to aid in understanding the usual pattern of functional loss and in planning for further support. The sections that follow on early, moderate, or severe stages of disease provide more examples to further understand these different stages and the changes they bring.

---

* Reisberg, B. Functional Assessment Staging (FAST). *Psychopharmacology Bulletin*. 1988;24: 653–659.

**TABLE 1.1** FAST Scale of Dementia Progression

| STAGE | DESCRIPTION | COMMON FUNCTIONAL FEATURES |
|---|---|---|
| 1 | Normal adult | No reported or perceived difficulties |
| 2 | Normal older adult | Complains of forgetting location of objects<br><br>Subjective word-finding difficulties |
| 3 | Early dementia | Decreased job function evident to coworkers<br><br>Difficulty traveling to new locations<br><br>Decreased organizational capacity (reported by self or others) |
| 4 | Mild dementia | Decreased ability to perform complex tasks (e.g., planning dinner for guests), handling finances (forgetting to pay bills), difficulty shopping |
| 5 | Moderate dementia | Requires assistance in choosing proper clothing to wear for the day, season, occasion |
| 6a* | Moderately severe dementia | Difficulty putting on clothing properly without assistance |
| 6b* | | Unable to bathe properly (e.g., difficulty adjusting water temperature) |
| 6c* | | Inability to handle mechanics of toileting (e.g., forgets to flush, does not wipe properly or properly dispose of tissue) |
| 6d | | Urinary incontinence, occasional or more frequent |
| 6e | | Fecal incontinence, occasional or more frequent |

**TABLE 1.1** (*continued*)

| STAGE | DESCRIPTION | COMMON FUNCTIONAL FEATURES |
|-------|-------------|----------------------------|
| 7a | Severe dementia | Ability to speak limited to approximately a half-dozen words or fewer, in the course of an average day or an intensive interview |
| 7b | | Speech ability limited to the use of a single intelligible word in an average day or the course of an interview |
| 7c | | Ambulatory ability lost (cannot walk without personal assistance) |
| 7d | | Ability to sit up without assistance lost (e.g., the individual will fall over if there are no lateral rests on chair) |
| 7e | | Loss of ability to smile |
| 7f | | Loss of ability to hold head up |

*Occasionally or more frequently over the past weeks.

## The Earlier Stages

In the early stages of dementia, functional loss is seen as difficulty navigating and planning work and social settings or as difficulty coming up with words to express feelings or meaning. Still, most individuals are able to live independently with minimal or no outside support.

## The Middle Stages

In the mid-stages of dementia, which can last anywhere from 1 to 15 years, individuals require assistance to remain independent. The assistance may be as minimal as reminders to take medication, but it may be more substantial with hands-on assistance needed for preparing meals, bathing, or dressing. Changes in personality or mood, poor judgment in clothing choices, difficulties navigating while driving or walking, or other safety factors may emerge. Caregivers are often familiar with this stage, because it is characterized by a push/pull with the individual who has dementia in an effort to balance independence with care assistance. That balance is not always easy to find. Many individuals and their care partners will recognize the *desire* to drive, but the individual with dementia may lack the understanding that this choice is no longer safe. This is one example of tiptoeing around the loss of independence on the fuzzy continuum to end-stage disease.

## The Later Stages

The transition to the final stages is difficult to spot at first. The final stages are known for the loss of ability to fully engage with the environment. This stage may be confusing for family members, as "good" days with glimmers of independence and function are interspersed with "bad" days that require assistance for safety or to avoid frustration. One family member questioned why her father was able to talk about the weather, smile at his grandchild crawling across the floor, and enjoy his strawberry shortcake dessert but could not toilet successfully. She was confused by the transitioning, with the retention of some abilities while others were lost. This mix of function made recognizing the transition to late stages difficult. In the late stages, *most* days can be described as the individual with dementia talking very little, showing little emotion or engagement (including facial response to the happenings around them), or being irritated with whatever is going on.

Full-time care assistance and supervision is required for most basic functions. In the transition from mid- to final stages, helping with bathing and selecting clothes increases to performing the bathing and dressing of your family member. Before the final stages, your relative may have been able to grab a sandwich or follow directions to heat up something in the microwave. In late stages, the meal must be set out and ready to eat, and, even then, it may be forgotten or your family member may need help with using utensils to eat. All walks and exercise must be supervised, because the risk of falling becomes a daily concern. Using the bathroom moves from a suggestion to a timed event that is met with resistance or the need to clean and change soiled clothing.

Communication becomes limited. Your family member may still be talking, but it may become more difficult to interpret what he or she is trying to communicate. The use of words becomes limited, imperfect, inadequate, and repetitive. Conversations may focus on only one old story. Your relative may use the same joke or social norm over and over to finagle out of an awkward situation, such as not knowing the answer to a simple question or the name of the familiar-looking person across the table. "What am I, Scrooge in the *Christmas Carol*? Isn't every day Christmas day if you're of the right mind?" would quip one of my favorite patients when asked to name the day or season during a routine mental status exam—the answer he gave every time on every visit.

These changes depict the beginnings of the late stages of Alzheimer disease and related dementias. The individual continues to decline to the end stages when talking stops, eating is accompanied by choking or appetite is gone, and walking is no longer possible. Most days are spent in a chair or a bed, and the individual must be lifted to avoid falling. The transition may seem gradual when you are involved in the care on a daily basis but is more obvious when a person is seen occasionally or intermittently. I did not always recognize the slip in my mom's function, but the changes would register when I saw my sister's reaction on one of her cross-country visits. Visits from others also calibrated my understanding that Alzheimer disease was marching on to its finale in my mom, as it does in everyone.

## ACCEPTING THE PROGRESSION OF THE DISEASE
### • *John's Story* •

John moved in with his son and daughter-in-law, Bart and Inga, when he transitioned from mild to a moderate stage of a mixed dementia. The move was triggered by several fender benders and parking "bumps." Although everyone knew that John would be isolated without a car, it was no longer safe for him to drive. Bart and Inga converted part of their house into an in-law apartment, and John puttered around the house, doing yard work and relishing the handyman jobs Inga asked him to perform. When the family ate dinner together, John would report how he had fixed a hinge, fertilized the garden, or picked the best tomato. Bart and Inga shared stories of their coworkers and their days at work. The family time together was peaceful and warm. But as John's dementia progressed, he lost the initiative to bathe and ensuring good hygiene became a struggle. Inga coached Bart in approaches to prepping baths beforehand and to firmly and gently encouraging John. In turn, Bart was now able to assist John in bathroom activities. However, without realizing it, Bart was spending more and more time helping John with his activities of daily living— those things we all need to do for basic self-care, such as eating, bathing, and dressing.

Bart's employment became less stable, and he and Inga decided to live on one income to decrease stress in the household and to accommodate John's growing physical needs. With each change, the family adapted to a new routine. But once Bart was home full time with John, Bart failed to notice John's continued cognitive and functional declines as well as the stresses caused by the increased daily care needs. John slept more in the day and was up and wandered at night. He began to urinate in trash cans and sinks. He sustained several injuries from falls. Inga recognized John's transition to the end stages of dementia and spoke with Bart about the need to alter their approach to his care. Bart, having been caught up in John's day-to-day care, resisted the idea. Inga insisted that Bart and John visit me for an objective assessment. My confirmation of Inga's impressions brought tears to Bart's eyes as he acknowledged his father's journey had entered a new phase. I knew Bart understood when his questions shifted from how could *he* keep John safe on his feet to how could *we* accommodate John's inability to walk safely? As hard as this last transition was for Bart to accept, it was a road to another level of peace.

---

## WHEN FAMILY MEMBERS LOSE
## THEIR VOICE TO DEMENTIA

In the late stages of dementia, the family member no longer has the mental capacity to make decisions, neither the big life-and-death decisions nor the little day-to-day decisions. By all means, we should continue to listen to our relative, for this loss of voice is not consistent, universal, or complete. In fact, we may need to listen ever more carefully, paying attention to nonverbal cues and verbal utterances for signs and signals that can indicate what is really wanted and needed. We should always make sure to listen, all the way to the end, and remain on constant alert so that we can respect and honor those messages that do come through.

Because dementia may impair judgment and change personality, it may also impair our family member's voice. This means our family member may not be able to clearly express what he or she wants or needs. Most of us may not want a bath when the air is cold, but if we've soiled ourselves, we would logically opt for the bath in cold air to avoid the odor and possible infection from unclean skin. Although our relative with dementia may express an opinion, caregivers need to look for the real message lurking behind the stated one. For example, a simple refusal to bathe may really mean, "I don't want to be cold." If the cold is addressed, the bath may not be rejected. Of course, if someone is offered juice or milk, preferences such as these can be easily ascertained and are of limited consequence. Another example is deciding what to wear on a cold, blustery day. An inappropriate selection may need some changes to ensure that the person is kept comfortably warm in bad weather.

We also need to recognize that the need for help in making decisions arises over and over, day in and day out. I am reminded of a children's book about math in which the child stated he doesn't need math as he will never use it. The rest of the book shows the boy realizing that math is all around him, even overwhelming him. Daily decisions, at times, may also become overwhelming when assisting someone with dementia, unless you are adequately prepared to make them.

---

## MAKING DECISIONS FOR ANOTHER
### • *Alicia and Ray's Story* •

Alicia and Ray were married only five years when I met them. This was the second marriage for each, although they had known each other as family friends. They were happy and in love, enjoying freedom, travel, and fun after caring for their former spouses, both of whom had died of cancer-related illnesses. Within the last year, Alicia had begun repeatedly asking the same questions and misplacing objects. Ray reported the real trouble started a few months ago when Alicia was hospitalized for a stomach illness and "just went crazy."

Alicia's son described delirium that prolonged her hospital stay and resulted in the need for additional medication. Plus, Alicia had a substantial loss in cognition and function after the hospitalization. Alicia and Ray came to me for a diagnosis and advice on how to cope with the new changes. After confirming Alicia's diagnosis of dementia and stabilizing or eliminating all unnecessary medications, Alicia's function did not markedly improve. Ray took charge of "everything," and it overwhelmed him. Ray fretted over what Alicia wore because her choices were not appropriate for the weather. He guided her food choices to avoid the swings between constipation and diarrhea that were common since Alicia's stomach situation. When he noticed that Alicia seemed fatigued,

Ray would urge naps but then wake her quickly so that the nap wouldn't interfere with her sleep at night. He insisted on exercise so that her blood pressure and pulse remained stable. Alicia and Ray's story highlights the host of care decisions that may need to be made—decisions that may seem never ending without a sense of balance and perspective. Alicia's son was more concerned with decisions about socialization and long-term plans. But Ray couldn't even contemplate long-term planning because he was so anxious about the numerous, ongoing daily decisions.

---

## THE CARE PARTNER'S PROCESS OF LETTING GO

### End-of-Life Decisions Will Be Needed

So how do we prepare to let go? Letting go can be approached mindfully and deliberately or the disease process and inevitability of death can carry us to the end without preparation. Taking a palliative approach to care in the terminal states of disease improves quality and quantity of life and diminishes caregiver stress. A frame of reference helps deliberation on end-of-life choices: a balance of prolonging life or prolonging death. Most favor goals to prolong life if quality of life can be maintained, but what if that is not possible? Prolonging death is stated in the negative, but put differently, are we allowing for a natural death? The default of the medical system is to prolong life regardless of unstated goals or quality of life. To opt for a different approach, patients or family members must ask for alternatives.

Family members and loved ones are upset with themselves, one another, or the health care system as they wrestle with the amount of care being delivered. Is it too little? Too much? Questions of "Am I causing her death?" or "Am I causing his suffering?" are common. Advanced dementia lasts, on average, a few months to three years, ultimately resulting in death. All medications, procedures, and approaches should be questioned from a new lens, rather than from the prevention or treatment focus common in early to moderate stages. Once the disease progresses to the late stages, as in cancer, the shift in focus to a palliative approach begins.

## Decisions about End-of-Life Care for Another

So how can we prepare to make choices? Because decisions in dementia care are usually made with the input of many family members, considering information from several perspectives allows those making the decisions to learn from multiple angles. It may be helpful to consider understanding letting go from the physiologic aspects of dementia, the emotional aspects of attachment to our family member, or the spiritual aspects of death and dying—the brain, heart, and soul of our decisions.

## The Physical Changes

Dementia is a terminal disease, although it is commonly seen mostly as a chronic state because the progression to death lasts, on average, 3 to 12 years. It is a progressive, degenerative disorder, similar to amyotrophic lateral sclerosis (Lou Gehrig disease) in that respect. Progressive indicates the disease marches forward without cure or remission. Degenerative indicates the loss of function, in this case in the brain, which serves as the control center for the body. As the brain progressively degenerates, the brain's cells are no longer able to make the chemicals, called neurotransmitters, that are used for communication between nerve cells. When cells are not being communicated with, they die. We see this loss of communication among different areas of the brain in functional consequences, such as the loss of ability to remember, speak, move efficiently and safely, or swallow. In Alzheimer dementia, abnormal deposits (called beta-amyloid plaques and neurofibrillary tangles) are found in the brain. These abnormal deposits are typical of the disease, but their importance is still unclear.

Predicting when the disease has progressed to near death is not exact in dementia, but certain observations can help estimate the timing. Information that guides hospice eligibility may also guide in understanding when the end of life is nearing. When the loss of ability to talk, walk, eat, toilet, and hold up the head is accompanied by repeated infections, skin breakdown, or loss in weight, the end of life is nearing. Little research is available to clearly address whether treating infections or providing assistance with feeding will help maintain life, but early findings suggest there is no difference in survival by doing so. So why suffer the side effects of these treatments or procedures? With this knowledge, families may understand that a focus on the *comfort* of the individual may be a better choice than treatment of an acute infection or worrying about weight loss.

## The Emotional Changes

There is a host of information on dealing with grief, but what about the period *before* grief? Because dementia often brings changes in personality, family members often start grieving before death. We spend a good deal of time handling—or not handling—emotional aspects of living and caring for someone with dementia. The time and energy to assist our family member adapt to and cope with dementia may seem all encompassing. Caregiving takes its toll. Caregivers may ignore their own health concerns and deal with depression and anxiety more than similarly aged non-caregivers. Preparing to let go must then be dealt with from this even more difficult state of less energy and depleted self-care.

What can help when the glass is half-empty? Curiosity, or perhaps broadening perspective, may help. Can you consider letting go from new angles or ideas to assist in your decisions? Can you question the difficult emotions that may accompany making decisions that affect the life and death of your relative? Feeling stuck or blocked in choices may arise from firmly held beliefs that do not allow for progress.

The discussions among my siblings regarding my mother's care were helpful, as we shared our emotional attitudes and how these beliefs translated to our opinions for her care. One sibling felt Mom should have had limited therapies from the beginning, because he highly valued mental capabilities and couldn't imagine she would want to live with less than her full mental capacity. Another sibling simply couldn't imagine ever stopping therapies. Because our beliefs were so different, we needed to explore one another's thought processes, which opened us to a number of valid ways to approach letting go and allowed us to reflect more deeply on what my mother may have chosen if she were able to tell us.

Ask questions to explore and challenge your own beliefs. Use the assistance of a therapist. Use tools known to help with personal growth, such as meditation and journaling. Support groups focusing on Alzheimer disease may expose you to ideas not previously considered. I tried many tools, including therapy, meditation, and journaling. Each became indispensable, helping me cope or illuminating a previously held belief that had me stuck in a repetitive and unhealthy thought pattern. When you're bothered by others challenging the difficult decisions you've made, ask yourself if they may be right. They may not be, but exposure to another idea may release the tension around a decision and allow you to be more confident in your choice.

---

## CHALLENGING A THOUGHT PROCESS TO EXPAND EMPATHY AND UNDERSTANDING

### • Kerry's Story •

A wonderful, caring daughter, Kerry cried and stated her brother had accused her of "killing" their mother with her care decisions. Kerry was hurt, defensive, and unhappy with her brother's words. I asked her to reflect on whether her brother's statements were true, to take the time to sit in his place and look at her mother from his eyes. She looked pensively out the window as she evaluated their mother's situation from her brother's perspective. A smile gradually crept across her face and her shoulders lowered. She softened to his concerns that the family was "giving up" their mother.

Kerry knew she was handling her mother's care as her mother would have wanted. She was not killing her mother but allowing for her natural death. She could now explain this more clearly to her brother and was confident in answering and addressing his concerns about what their mother wanted and that her comfort and care was everyone's top concern.

---

If you feel stuck in a cycle of repetitive thoughts or all of your thoughts are full of despair, it may be time to seek professional guidance to assist you in coping with being the decision maker in someone's life. Depression and anxiety commonly accompany caregiving. Counselors or social workers may assist with framing context or perspective on decisions and sorting out whether depression is interfering with or complicating decision making.

## The Spiritual Considerations

Losing a family member is one of the largest stressors in life. It is pain that does not leave but is assimilated into our being and life experience. The alternative side of times of pain is what opens us to personal or spiritual growth. Countless memoirs of transformation come from experiences of tragedy and loss. Illness can open us to community that can help us in loss—loss of the personality or loss of the person. Faith, or a teaching in Buddhism or mindfulness practice called nonattachment, can help us deal with the progression of the disease and the inevitable death. Prayer or meditation can help us transcend the daily routine of caregiving or turmoil of difficult decisions. Seeking the community of an organized religion, building the support of similar-minded spiritual journeyers, and learning from the timeless wisdom of spiritual leaders or from the speeches and writings of philosophers and poets can all be used to prepare us as our relative leaves this physical world.

Spiritual guides and clergy, much like counselors and social workers, may aid in addressing end-of-life decisions. We may be searching for answers, comfort, and confidence in decisions that trigger concerns such as "Am I playing God?" or "How can I live with myself once I make this decision?" The perspective and contemplation of someone who considers these questions often and discusses them with many families can be very helpful. Each of us has our own values, but spiritual leaders and clergy are trained in value assessment and discussion. I have joined the chaplain of an inpatient palliative care service in family meetings to discuss decisions for end-of-life care. Many times, I have sensed palpable relief fill a room as the chaplain gently guides difficult discussions, interjecting opinions and questions to find a reflective, peaceful, and touching resolution.

## CONSIDERING THE WHOLE PERSON
### • *Janet's Story* •

Janet was in her late 80s, confined to bed, and noncommunicative from her late-stage dementia. She lived in a skilled nursing facility and had been sent to the hospital for the third time in three months, this time for evaluation of a fever. She had a urinary tract infection and was dehydrated and very sleepy. Her daughter, Elaine, was constantly at her mother's bedside and, according to the staff, had "too many questions and too high expectations." The resident in charge of Janet's care asked me, "What does Elaine expect us to do for her mother?" The nurses requested a palliative care consult to ease the tension between Elaine and the house staff, because they felt the conflict interfered with care goals and added to Janet's suffering.

Katy, the hospital chaplain, offered to meet with me, the house staff, and Elaine. As expected, Elaine came with a list of questions and the house staff was armed with answers. But all conversations focused on medicine, not people. Katy listened and watched. I asked Elaine to tell us about Janet as a younger woman, before she was too sick to speak, before dementia took her voice. Elaine's voice would catch as she described a vibrant, loving woman and the information she had gleaned about Janet's wishes from memories of long ago conversations. Katy listened and watched. I and the house staff reported on Elaine's prognosis in light of weight loss and repeated infections and hospitalizations. Katy continued to listen and watch. Elaine asked what would happen if we stopped care. I explained the probable course from a medical perspective. Elaine looked to Katy. Katy could see that Elaine was really asking about her mother the woman, not her mother the patient. Katy said, "I do not know, but we can talk more about it." Elaine relaxed and said "I would appreciate that."

Katy and Elaine went for a walk and discussed Elaine's concerns about her mother's prognosis, care plan, and life. Katy knew Elaine needed time, an ear, and a large dose of human compassion—something not always offered in the medical environment. Once Elaine felt heard and supported, she was no longer as confrontational. She began to listen in a way that she had not before. The house staff responded, better appreciating Janet as a more complete woman and better understanding Elaine as a supportive and caring daughter who was confused and feeling alone in the medical world. Elaine and the house staff began to lean on one another for information about Janet so that all felt better about Janet's care. In the next few days, Elaine concluded that being in the hospital was not benefiting Janet, and Janet returned to the skilled nursing facility for care directed more toward comfort than cure.

---

## GOALS OF CARE

All decisions, including avoiding decisions, are decisions. In the United States, avoiding a medical decision results in receiving aggressive medical care. But there is an alternative—deliberating on the choices available; seeking advice and guidance from health care professionals, family, friends, social workers, and spiritual guides; and deciding on a path forward. In a chronic and progressive disease such as Alzheimer dementia, a cure is not available. The goals of care are tailored to the individual based on the stage of dementia, and the expected outcomes may vary.

---

### HAVING CLEAR GOALS OF CARE
#### • Maybel's Story •

A dear friend sought my counsel on several occasions regarding if and when to hospitalize his mother, Maybel. When Maybel was in the moderate stages of dementia, she became acutely short of breath, feverish, and difficult to awaken. Jon was concerned and confused about the next best action. He and his family had clear goals of care for end of life, not wanting to prolong Maybel's life when the disease had progressed to late stages. But was Maybel at this stage? Jon and I discussed the specific aspects of his mother's condition to make the best choice for her. Jon dreaded sending Maybel to the hospital because she had become confused and combative during a recent hospitalization for hip surgery, and she had never completely regained her previous level of function and cognition. We discussed how a transfer to the hospital could help Maybel (oxygen, intravenous antibiotics, and intravenous hydration), also acknowledging that there were risks (delirium, potential for unwanted aggressive intervention such as intubation, exposure to other infections) in her current state.

Maybel was walking and eating well, but she was beginning to transition to the later stages of dementia with less meaningful conversation, less awareness of her surroundings, and more time sleeping. If Maybel developed swallowing difficulty, the family did not want another hospitalization or treatment of recurrent pneumonia. Jon questioned whether Maybel was choking or whether there could be another explanation for her symptoms. I thought this episode of shortness of breath followed a common cold that had likely progressed to pneumonia.

With this insight, Jon chose hospitalization. The family remained at Maybel's bedside day and night to ensure that the limits on her care (such as no intubation) were honored, to minimize delirium by having someone recognizable present each time she opened her eyes, and to prevent Maybel from climbing out of bed unassisted and falling. Maybel did well and returned home to a good quality of life for another two years. Understanding the goals of Maybel's care—to manage reversible conditions that were not the result of progression of her dementia diagnosis—assisted the family to make the complex series of decisions.

---

## Disease Progression May Change Goals of Care

Focusing on goals of care takes the sting out of many decisions that will be required as your relative transitions through the final stage of dementia. Goals of care can be used as a compass in a dark night, when you feel you've lost your way. Goals of care will be your map. Reviewing and revisiting the goals of care regularly help all involved see the best way forward. Understanding what can be expected is useful knowledge when one stands at these decision points.

Do you (or did your family member) value life over comfort? Does this change depending on the stage of disease you are in? Is being able to meaningfully interact more important than comfort? Is being awake more important than being comfortable from pain or anxiety? How would these decisions change as you (or family members) move through a disease and as you approach the end of what the medical community can offer for prolongation of life? Knowing the different options available will help you decide on the care for your relative that you are most comfortable with—the care that your relative previously expressed or that you think your relative would want—rather than allowing, by default, the medical community to decide as your family lets go of the physical life of the person with dementia.

▶ Dementia is a chronic, progressive, and degenerative disease. The progression is unpredictable, and there is no known cure so the result, ultimately, is death.

▶ Later stages of dementia typically occur for months to approximately three years.

▶ Hallmarks of later stages are loss of ability to toilet, talk, walk, and engage in meaningful ways with the environment.

▶ Decision making, for medical and nonmedical issues, in later stages of dementia must be integrated into the care provided by family.

▶ Care partners require emotional preparation to adapt to decision making for another.

▶ Understanding the late stages of dementia may help care partners prepare to participate in care for a relative.

▶ Establishing and frequently reevaluating goals of care aid in determining action at the multiple decision points in the care of a relative with dementia.

ACTION PLAN

▶ Keep a journal documenting the functional status of your family member. Use instrumental activities of daily living in early stages (shopping, housekeeping, accounting, food preparation, managing medications, ability to use telephone, ability to drive or use transportation) and basic activities of daily living as the dementia progresses (bathing, grooming, dressing, toileting, transferring or walking safely, eating). In the final stages, also note speaking (are words limited, speaking rare?) and sleeping (are the hours in bed or naps increasing?). The journal, if updated monthly, will assist in seeing the progression and adapting to changing needs.

▶ Make a list of people who can be used as resources. Suggestions include a friend who has helped a family member living with dementia, clergy, physician, therapist, and housekeeper. When you're faced with multiple decisions, is there anyone on the list who you can call for advice or assistance?

▶ Begin to explore your opinions about care with advanced dementia. Journal on your thoughts and questions. What are your core beliefs about death? Your experience? Do you think of death as always bad? Can you imagine when death may be preferable to life? As you contemplate your questions, review the physical changes that accompany dementia, the emotional strain of making decisions for another, and the spiritual aspects of facing death.

▶ Develop goals of care for your family member for now. Imagine his or her life in six months or one year—what may change the goals? Consider a course before the crisis occurs so that you can ask questions at the next medical visit or be prepared at the time of an emergency visit to the health care system.

## ADDITIONAL READING AND RESOURCES

▶ The Alzheimer's Association

This website (https://www.alz.org/) provides reputable educational material on Alzheimer disease and related dementia, resources for caregiving, and updates on research and policy relating to dementia.

▶ *Being Mortal: Medicine and What Matters in the End*, by Atul Gawande, MD

Dr. Gawande explores the common approach of the health care system to disease in the beginning of the twenty-first century. The book has insights into an approach to care that acknowledges mortality, including a discussion of mortality when faced with the condition of Alzheimer dementia.

▶ *The 36-Hour Day: A Family Guide to Caring for People Who Have Alzheimer Disease, Other Dementias, and Memory Loss*, 6th ed., by Nancy L. Mace and Peter V. Rabins

This book is an excellent source of complete information on dementia. It includes a discussion of the causes of dementia, in-depth information on earlier stages, and many suggestions for caregivers.

▶ *The Places That Scare You: A Guide to Fearlessness in Difficult Times*, by Pema Chodron

This book, written by a Buddhist nun, provides a guide to approaching difficult situations from a place of love and compassion, rather than from a place of fear. The approach acknowledges the struggles in life and invites the reader to explore these experiences from a place of joy, strength, and courage.

# Preparing to Let Go: Emotions of Caring

Care partners need to acknowledge their emotions and find strategies to cope with these myriad feelings. Care partners also may experience different emotions at different times—in the context of beginning to let go or when beginning to honor the process of the death that accompanies the diagnosis of dementia. But before we can let go, we must prepare for the emotions involved in the process.

---

### DEALING WITH A SPECTRUM OF EMOTIONS
#### • *The Kenny Family Story* •

I visited my mother daily, sometimes with my daughter or son in tow, sometimes alone. We spent time playing bingo with the other residents of her assisted living facility; my daughter was honored to be selected to verify the winner of each game, checking the card of the triumphant for accuracy. My son and mother would walk the hallway or the garden, weaving into each other, trying to trip each other up to elicit a smile. We would all sing "A Bicycle Built for Two," and my kids would roll their eyes as my mother and I hammed it up together.

When I visited alone, I would sit forehead-to-forehead with my mother, whispering my fears about life—that one child was being picked on, that I was concerned my tenure may not be granted, or that I wasn't doing a good job balancing work and family. And then it all began to change. My mom's face became less animated and her eyes became flatter. She began coughing violently, gasping, spewing, and turning blue at the most random moment. The kids visited less often, and incidents like these would result in my daughter becoming quiet and begging to go home as soon as everyone's heart rates had returned to normal after another successful Heimlich maneuver. My son had to catch his grandmother from falling on their walks, no longer a fun and playful diversion escaping my watchful eye. As my mom's disease progressed, no more bingo, no more walks, no more singing. Only restless squirming at my stories. My emotions ran the gamut from love, joy, and appreciation of the childhood memories of a storytelling, piecrust-baking mother to sadness, confusion, and exhaustion at a new reality of a mother with distant stares devoid of emotion or flashes of anger, restlessness, or frustration.

These emotions I could understand, feel, and allow to move through me with laughter and tears. Well . . . honestly, I could once I had sought the help of a wonderful therapist and began to meditate regularly. The hardest were the ugly emotions I was feeling—the worry, guilt, boredom, anger, and resentment. At times, I felt schizophrenic: grateful one moment for the time I had with my mother, and guilty and worthless the next that I had not done enough to care for her.

---

## LOSS AND CHANGED RELATIONSHIPS

As family members change and become less of the person we knew, we often feel lost and confused by our changing roles from that of partners or family members to caregivers for someone we don't always recognize. How can we remain angry at a father who neglected us as children, when the person sitting in front of us has lost his fists and fury? How can we feel tenderness toward a mother who baked for us and kissed our bruised knee, when that person is now spitting and cursing at us? How do we face the constant decisions we need to make—and then defend—when challenged by family, the health care system, friends, or neighbors who may not be aware of or understand the complex circumstances that factored into those decisions?

## Ambiguous Loss

Some of the difficulty with care partnering with someone living with dementia is the type of loss. Pauline Boss, PhD, describes some of the emotions associated with care as "ambiguous loss." The difficulty is that the person is physically present but at times psychologically gone—the relationship you've always known is altered. Dr. Boss describes difficulty arising because there is no closure. The usual outcomes we expect when someone is with us or has left us are not present, because the situation is neither. Many emotions, many that are unusual or have not previously been experienced, are often stirred in care partnering with one with dementia. There have been adjustments to new roles, such as becoming the caregiver to a parent or the dominant spouse when previously roles had been different.

Adjusting to the primary decision-maker role for another adult can be quite difficult. Making a decision for oneself can be challenging enough because of the circumstances but often "feels" right because the responsibility for living with the outcome affects mostly yourself. Choosing for another is more difficult because understanding the "right" choice can be both complex and varied. Adjusting to this ambiguous loss is usually hard won. And then it is time to adjust again, to let go of the next ambiguous state. The territory of emotional uncertainty is waded into again. The time of letting go allows us to continue to practice what the journey with Alzheimer disease or a related dementia has demanded from us all—the ability to change and adapt and enhance our resiliency.

---

### DIFFERING SIBLINGS, DIFFERING PERSPECTIVES
#### • *The Olsens' Story* •

I met with Coleen and Connie to discuss their mother, Corky, and her progression with dementia. Coleen arrived on time and apologized for her sister's tardiness. She seemed both embarrassed and frustrated and admitted she wasn't sure her sister would even show up. Connie arrived 10 minutes later. In contrast to Coleen's plump appearance and conservative dress, Connie was thin, haggard, and dressed in sparkles. She did not respond to either my greeting or extended hand but pursed her lips and tersely said, "Just keep going wherever you were."

Although the sisters sat side by side, they were as far from each other as possible—complete opposites. We began a long discussion beginning with their mother's diagnosis and the course her dementia had taken. Coleen described her and her mother's emotional responses to changes over the years, while Connie sat stone-faced, offering no information on her feelings or perspective, even when I asked directly if she had anything to add. When I asked them if Corky had given them any guidance on how she might want to approach end of life, Coleen said that her parents never talked of death or dying when they were young or when other family members died. I counseled that these types of situations often unearth difficult emotions in those who now need to make decisions for their family member without the benefit of knowing their family member's opinion or wishes. Coleen began to cry, while Connie's face stiffened further.

I asked Connie first for her input on the next best step; she deferred to her sister. Coleen said she understood that her mother's time was limited regardless of what could be done, but she still didn't want to lose her. She said, "It seems wrong, but selfishly, I want my mother to be here, even though I can see that she is suffering." Connie chimed in for the first time. "I don't want to see her suffer any longer and that is all she is doing. She is suffering." There was a long pause while the sisters looked at each other. Connie then looked squarely at me and said, "I don't want to lose my mother either, but she is suffering so much. She wouldn't want this." I thanked her for her candidness and looked to Coleen. Coleen said, "I agree Mom is suffering. I thought I was holding onto hope she might get better, but now I see I just couldn't face losing her." We all agreed there is no good time to lose one's mother. After a few minutes of holding a place for these tender feelings, the sisters began to make decisions together for their mother with a goal of comfort and stopping suffering.

---

## THE GOOD

I learned to be present with my mother—it was uplifting and we found love, joy, happiness, and hope. It was amazing. I was lucky because I knew it was possible. I had seen other people do it. It was less ambiguous for me. The people I modeled my acceptance and approach after weren't unusual or saints (well . . . maybe they were, but not *all* the time). They were resilient. They adapted to what was thrown their way and looked for the best in it. And they found plenty. Myriad good emotions can come from partnering in care with someone who is dying from dementia. There is a host of good—*love, joy, gratitude, hope, and dreams.*

Many memoirs discuss the trials and tribulations of life and become tales of transformation. Myths and fairy tales are filled with the same. Joseph Campbell, an American mythologist, writer, and lecturer, best known for his work in comparative mythology and religion, discusses the heroic voyage archetype in *The Hero with a Thousand Faces.* Campbell describes a number of stages or steps along the hero's journey: an ordinary start, the call to enter an unusual world, task and trial either dealt with alone or in companionship, and if the hero survives, his or her reward—a great gift that results in discovery of important self-knowledge. I heard tales such as these from several people who cared for a spouse or a parent, and, although they were tired when the journey was over, these individuals emerged with a broader perspective, wiser, and gratified. I must say that this is also true of my journey accompanying my mother.

Of course I got it wrong several times along the way: I tussled with my siblings over differing opinions of approach to care. I snarled at paid care providers for not cleaning my mother's teeth or clothes or room just so. I snapped at my children to appreciate all they had when they asked for a tiny little thing on a day I felt I had nothing left to give. But I also slowed my life down enough to sit quietly in the same chair by a window with my mother day after day and watch a robin build and line a nest, lay eggs, hatch fledglings, and feed them until they flew away. This time of quieting my life down opened me to ask questions, to reevaluate my own life journey. I faced my rushed and impatient attitude toward others to reveal and finally understand that the issue was not them but me throwing a controlled temper tantrum.

In *Ten Thousand Joys and Ten Thousand Sorrows*, Olivia Ames Hoblitzelle describes her husband's (and her) thoughtful, mindful journey with Alzheimer disease. Their approach, based in a mindful practice, allowed for all the emotions of life. The joys and the sorrows. They lived completely. They acknowledged death as the natural ending to the disease. They did not shy away from any part of the full range of emotions they faced. Because roles change and losses occur during this unique disease process, we may inadvertently ignore the fullness of the experience. Assisting someone in exiting this world and being the one who makes the last decisions will be fraught with many emotions and can be especially complex, because our relationship with the individual with dementia, with ourselves, and our (and their) beliefs about death and dying are intermixed.

---

## MAKING POSITIVE FAMILY CHANGES IN THE MIDST OF LIVING AND DYING WITH DEMENTIA
### • Ruby's Family's Story •

Ruby and her two daughters, Agnes and Thea, first came to see me when Ruby was in mid-stage dementia and her quality of life was abysmal from mouth pain. Ruby was living alone at the time and struggling to maintain herself. Agnes and Thea were concerned that their mother was miserable from pain, worried about the possibility of something ominous, such as an undiagnosed cancer. They brought me Ruby's medical records of several previous workups that established this was not a physical problem. Ruby was a strong matriarch and had retained many of her social skills and her controlling, even domineering, demeanor. Her daughters were both markedly different—Agnes was easygoing, down-to-earth, and relaxed, while Thea was dignified, formal, and reserved. They did not seem close on our first meeting but more the yin and yang to Ruby's presence.

After reviewing the case, I began a series of discussions with Ruby and her daughters. I thought the mouth pain was related to stress and possibly depression from managing life in the face of dementia. I recommended a change in living situation to support the deficits in Ruby's functioning while maintaining as much of her independence as possible. We would also try changing Ruby's medications to focus on the depression and anxiety rather than on the pain itself. Ruby was willing to give it a try, but Agnes and Thea appeared shocked. They wondered how could they possibly support their mother, the mother who ruled all worlds she stepped into? They rallied and adapted. They decided their mother would move in with each of them for three-month blocks of time. I cautioned them about preserving their own lives and life balance as best they could. The sisters worked out respite breaks for each other in the middle of their three-month blocks.

They marveled at the positive transformation in their mother, once she relaxed in their homes, relieved from the stress of running a household herself. And the sisters grew in other ways. Ruby loved the role of pampered queen and could be quite difficult. The sisters learned boundaries with their queen in order to live peacefully with their own families—not always easy as Ruby retained her powerful social skills. But the sisters dug deep to find power of their own, opening up to each other and learning from the other's strengths. Their families grew together.

When they came in for yearly checkups, I heard tales of Ruby's trials and triumphs, losses and surrenders. And I heard tales of the trials and triumphs of the sisters as well. Agnes became stronger and more self-assured. Thea learned to roll with the punches. Ruby thrived in her own way, progressively losing function but not her dignity. Agnes and Thea learned to "read" Ruby and know when a behavior was likely an expression of stress; this allowed them to explore ways to provide more support until the behavior was managed. They understood that the transition between houses would become more difficult as Ruby's dementia progressed, but that the respite for themselves and their families was a needed priority. Agnes and Thea spent time in each other's homes to assist in the transition periods. They mindfully adapted to each physical and functional loss, and they consciously built joy and happiness into their days. They avoided burnout. They avoided personal loss of health and minimized loss of finances. They were open to a positive experience in the midst of daily challenges. On each visit, they asked for information about what was likely to come next and how they might prepare. They had become an open and joyful team, a beautiful example of a family coming together and growing together.

Agnes, Thea, and I wept together when it was time for Ruby to enter hospice. They thanked me for accompanying them on their journey and said honestly that their mother living with dementia had been a true gift to their family. Ruby died eight months later, surrounded by a loving and tight-knit family.

---

I learned several lessons from Ruby's family. They practiced several strategies that helped them maintain their joy, happiness, and sanity during their journey with dementia. And their approach was multifaceted. They gathered knowledge of dementia itself. In this way, they lived well in the present with Ruby but prepared for changes that were likely coming. By anticipating these changes, they did not resist or fight against them. The sisters continued to acknowledge Ruby's longtime personality traits and the changes in her personality that were likely due to dementia. Distinguishing the differences helped them build boundaries (when Ruby was abusing her queen status) or adapt to changes caused by the disease (when Ruby couldn't manage the simplest task).

They acknowledged they needed each other to get through this. By placing boundaries around some of Ruby's behaviors, they were able to preserve her dignity as well as their own. They allowed some of Ruby's queen behavior but did not tolerate when she crossed the line and became mean. They looked for joyful practices and found ways to incorporate happiness in their days. They maintained family rituals and celebrations. They practiced gratitude daily. They maintained their hopes and dreams, for their mother (daily moments of joy and a good death), for themselves (daily moments of joy with their mother and their families, personal growth, peace), and for their families (wonderful memories of a family supporting their mother/grandmother).

## THE BAD

There is an abundance of literature on the difficulties that may accompany the journey of someone with dementia and their caregivers. We are now focusing on caregivers as they acknowledge and accept some of the emotions that accompany caregiving and the need to take on decision making for their family member. These decisions may become even more complicated when they involve complex and sensitive end-of-life choices.

Part of the difficulty in dealing with emotions may come from physical issues. Certain realities do not accompany other conditions, such as sleepless nights, or if they do, they seem mostly limited. For example, most infants do eventually sleep through the night—though I remember doubting this when my children were about three months old. Following on the heels of a toddler is a stage that lasts only a year or so, until these youngsters learn about safety and not to wander off. The disease process in dementia is unpredictable, and changes such as wandering, day and night shifts, and hallucinations or impulsive outbursts do not develop on a typical schedule. So issues of physical and mental exhaustion and time for privacy are often paramount, thus leading to what many consider some of the "bad" emotions or conditions—confusion, grieving, loneliness, isolation, and frustration—and may progress to the "ugly" emotions or conditions —worry, guilt, anger, resentment, and abuse.

---

## LEARNING TO CARE FOR ONESELF
### • Stephanie's Story •

Stephanie was a sweet, well-meaning woman in her mid-60s. She came to see me often, with complaints of aches and pains, sinus infections, hair loss, weight gain, twisted ankle, sore shoulder. She would be slumped in the chair when I entered the room but sat up straighter and straighter as we talked about her complaints. By the time she left the office, it was as if she were a plant that had just been watered after a drought. She would be humming and chatting gaily with the nursing and office staff. Stephanie cared for both her husband, who had early-onset dementia, and her mother, who had Alzheimer dementia. Stephanie admitted the only time she took for herself was making appointments to care for her own minor medical conditions. In the first few years, I encouraged her to take better care of herself, preserving her energy and balance so she could continue to care for her family. We discussed that her medical issues would escalate if she continued to lose sleep, eat only junk-on-the-run, and lift and twist without using proper technique.

And the time came. Stephanie was hospitalized with pneumonia, and her husband and mother needed to be placed in skilled nursing centers while she recovered. The episode scared Stephanie. Fortunately, her husband thrived at the facility, so she took the step to have him remain there, where she could visit him daily. Stephanie brought her mother home but arranged for her to attend a day program. She started to take some time for herself and began to build a group of friends, "so I have someone to travel with when my husband and my mother are gone." This allowed Stephanie to balance her support of her family with caring for herself. Her husband died three years later, and her mother about nine months after that. Stephanie grieved the loss of her family and her role as a caregiver, but she had a network of friends who supported her. The summer after her mother died, Stephanie went on a "girlfriends' weekend" to scrapbook and dance. She came back for an appointment with a sprained ankle, again. "This time it was from living it up. I know it's a re-injury of the first twist. I wouldn't give up either one—I am living a full life."

---

Stephanie found that isolation was adding to her burden of stress. She was brave to recognize that her husband was flourishing in an environment with more stimulation. She had the courage to explore new ways of coping. Dropping a rigid approach in the face of a constantly changing disease can open up new possibilities.

## Unresolved Family Issues

Another common scenario faced in caregiving is unresolved family issues. It may be difficult to care for an individual when the relationship may range, on the negative spectrum, from not close, to unaccepting, to hostile. At times, the anger and hurt or abuse from a marriage or childhood prevents individuals from taking direct care of the other person. Family members report that they fear they do not have the empathy and compassion for the individual who treated them so badly and fear they would retaliate with abuse or neglect. Having a family member live in a facility that provides the daily care is often the best option for a family in situations such as this. I've seen healing for the spouse or children when they witness the facility caregivers respond positively and in a caring manner to the individual who is living with and changed by dementia, allowing the spouse or children to look at their family member with fresh eyes, drop their resentments, feel compassion, and begin to forgive.

Similar emotions may accompany decision making with siblings who have held onto grudges from their youth or adulthood. Consciously deciding to let go of resentment or vengeance toward another who has harmed you in some way results in numerous health benefits, including improved sleep quality, blood pressure, and immune function and less stress and depression. Forgiveness does not mean condoning or forgetting the action, but realizing that holding onto the emotions and replaying the hurt causes repeated hurts, with ill effects on physical and mental health for the individual holding onto the hurt. Several strategies are used to foster the ability to forgive and to help modulate and reduce negative emotions (often a good idea for numerous situations for a caregiver). Strategies may include enhancing empathy, searching for the good in any situation, and acknowledging your feelings, either in person or through journaling. In *Just One Thing: Developing a Buddha Brain One Simple Practice at a Time*, Rick Hanson, PhD, a neuropsychologist at the Greater Good Science Center of the University of California, offers 50 small practices that can train your brain to enhance well-being.

---

### PUTTING THE PAST IN THE PAST
#### • The Roberts's Story •

Lillian was a tall, slight woman. She sat in a wheelchair, hands resting passively on the armrests, eyes drooping. When I greeted her, she looked up at me but said nothing, with her voice, eyes, or face. Her daughter, Lydia, sharply laughed and partly barked, "Well, *now* she's all meek and mild." When I asked about Lillian and her family, Lydia again laughed sharply. "Where do I begin? She won't sleep, she fights me at every turn, she won't talk except when she finds the perfect words to curse at me, and she won't move except when I find her halfway across a room when I do look away for a minute. I can't leave her, I have to do everything for her, and all I get in return is cursing and cross looks, spitting, and shouting. She's thin but strong when she fights. And she makes me do everything!"

When Lydia was done, she folded her arms *tightly* across her chest and set her jaw. I gently laid my hand on Lillian's arm while I directed my comments to Lydia. I told her I could hear the intense emotions in her words and that we would address that after she was able to tell me more about Lillian's medical history and course. If I could help them as a family understand what was happening, we could come up with a plan. When I acknowledged that this was an emotional time, Lydia rolled her eyes, but she also welled up with tears. It was a beginning.

Sorting out Lillian's medications to more successfully address pain so she could sleep and find some peace took several sessions. Lydia remained angry and upset for months. I worked with Lydia to help her understand dementia and accompanying behaviors; encouraged her to find support from family, a therapist, or a support group; and recommended several books that might help her find some joy in her time with her mother.

Our first positive encounter was nearly a year later when I entered the exam room to find Lydia flipping through a magazine, giggling while Lillian smiled. Lydia said, "Thought you'd never see this, did you?" I said it was a nice surprise. Lydia reported that things were much better at home. She understood the disease better and how to handle bad days, but she admitted that she was still so angry. Her therapist worked with her to understand that the anger toward her mother had never been dealt with from when she was a teen. "My therapist asked me how long I planned to keep taking this poison. My mother obviously doesn't remember that time anymore. The therapist helped me see we had both been doing the best we could at the time. And we are doing the best we can now. It helps me forgive myself when I have a less than perfect day, remembering she didn't always have the best days taking care of me while I was growing up, but she didn't hold it over me day after day. I think I've finally grown up."

---

I learned so much as a caregiver to my children and to my mother. One of my best friends has a daughter with autism. She said when her daughter was diagnosed and she was feeling distraught and unsure, a friend of hers relayed a story that she thinks of often and shares with others who are dealing with overwhelming situations. *A woman boards a plane for Paris, planning all the wonderful sights she'll see there. The food, the history, the language, the people, the culture. When the plane lands, she finds herself in Holland. After the initial shock that she is not where she thought she'd be, the woman has a choice: lament that she is not in Paris or explore the wonders of Holland.* My friend has a beautiful and full relationship with her daughter. This story was key in my developing a full and beautiful relationship with my "new and ever changing" mother. I know this story has helped many of my patients and their families.

## Strategies for Dealing with Difficult Emotions

Emotions and realities of isolation, confusion, despair, and sadness may creep into our lives, especially under the responsibility of caring for another. In a mindful practice, we learn to "welcome everything, push away nothing." This sounds difficult, but resisting an emotion can cause it to linger. Sit with an emotion or a feeling and watch it. It will be there, intense and palpable, but then it will pass. Breathe through it. Be curious about it. Does it remind you of another time you felt like this in your life? Where do you feel it—physically? Is it a pressure in your head, a rock in your gut, a quickening of your breath? That sensation will fall away as well. Once the emotion has passed, there is often relief and space to accept and think and plan. I found when I was experiencing worry or sadness or isolation, when I sat with the feeling, I could come to the present moment and realize "right now" I was fine, my mother was fine, my kids were fine. I would be calmer and think more clearly. I still didn't know the answer or the way forward, but for "right now" I was doing alright.

## THE UGLY

The emotions that pack a punch include worry, guilt, anger, and resentment, which may lead to depression or to abuse and exploitation.

We need to recognize depression if it begins. Studies have shown that caregiving puts an individual at higher risk for depression. How do you know if you are suffering from depression? Screens are available that may help you recognize whether you are depressed.

Ask yourself some questions:

- Do you have trouble sleeping?
- Do you feel sad or hopeless?
- Have you lost interest in usual activities?
- Do you feel guilty?
- Do you lack energy?
- Do you cry often or are you easily irritated?
- Have you lost or gained weight?
- Do you have trouble concentrating?
- Have you considered hurting yourself as an only way out of these feelings?

If you suspect you are depressed or some of these symptoms have been present for a few weeks, it is time to see a health care professional for confirmation and assistance. Therapists can provide a safe outlet and suggest readings or activities that will help you recover from depression and anxiety. Physicians can suggest medications if needed. Therapy in combination with medications can be very effective.

## Unchecked Negative Emotion May Lead to Abuse or Exploitation

If worry, anger, guilt, resentment, or depression is not addressed, these dark emotions may escalate to include abuse or exploitation. Abuse of older people comes in many guises. It can be physical (non-accidental use of force that results in pain or injury), emotional (intimidating or humiliating language or terrorizing and menacing behavior, including isolation), financial (including misuse of funds or the individual's signature to falsify legal documents, including wills), or sexual. The most common type of abuse in older people,

comprising approximately 50 percent of cases, is neglect or aban-
donment. One in five (20%) caregivers fear they will become violent
with an individual for whom they care, while studies show that 5–10
percent actually are physically abusive. Studies have further shown
that 40–60 percent of caregivers have been verbally abusive to their
family member. What puts so many caregivers at risk of becoming
abusive? Anxiety, depression, social isolation, and feeling burdened
are common causes, as is the family member with dementia demon-
strating verbal or physical aggression.

## Strategies to Counter Risk of Abuse

Knowing how common abuse is, we can understand that *we are all
at risk*. The importance of recognizing the risk is to put preventive mechanisms in place. Addressing our negative emotions is
paramount.

I will repeat the suggestion to speak with professionals.

Rick Hanson's *Just One Thing* gives several strategies to care for
yourself, enjoy life, build emotional strength, engage with the world,
and be at peace. Most of these strategies occur only in the mind, so
time away from the house is not required. Dr. Hanson recommends
practicing these strategies to build neural strength, much as you'd
build muscles with weight lifting.

Unfortunately, there is little research on preventing abuse in
older adults. It is unclear whether understanding the risks for abuse
is helpful to the caregiver to enhance awareness and prompt self-
control during a time of a trigger. A small study in England suggests
that providing caregivers with a manual that covers understanding
dementia and behaviors, accessing emotional support, changing un-
helpful thoughts, learning techniques for assertive communication,
planning for the future, and increasing pleasant activities can result
in less anxiety and depression for caregivers; however, abusive behavior did not change in this study, which may have been too small
to see this effect.

## Risk of Financial Exploitation

A final "ugly" emotion comes in the form of greed or exploitation. The most common individuals to misuse or exploit individuals are family members. They often justify the exploitation by their caregiving, but objective onlookers do not view the caregiving as optimal. For example, there have been instances of care intended to prolong life for the purpose of keeping pensions and housing stable, movement of resources to spouse's or children's accounts with the broken promise of providing stimulating day programs or enhanced in-home care, and respite that does not happen because of "limited funds." Individuals with dementia have lost their voice and ability to advocate for themselves. Health care professionals can report suspected abuse, but all too often limited resources dictate that only the most egregious cases are addressed.

Forensic studies suggest that prevention via limiting social isolation is the best way to protect a vulnerable older adult from financial exploitation. In a family, it is best if the individual involved with the financial responsibility has a secondary check. In my family, my brother would ask others for input on his decisions, both as a personal check on his moral compass (which wasn't required, but says so much) and to keep more than one person abreast of my mother's financial position as her condition deteriorated.

---

### RECOGNIZING EXPLOITATION
#### • *Andy and Brett's Story* •

Andy had a gregarious, take-the-world-by-storm personality when I met him about a year after his diagnosis with dementia. He felt confident that as the trials and tribulations of dementia struck, he would weather them with vigor and pluck. He admitted that he initially needed to deal with depression and anger but now desired to live—truly live—every day he could. He also planned to set out clear directives for how he wanted to limit care and let "nature take its course" when the disease progressed. We discussed his need for a durable power of attorney who would understand and agree to follow his plan of care.

He was in a second marriage with Brett, a woman 20 years his junior, and had already put all his assets in her name and named her durable power of attorney. However, now Andy had some misgivings as he confided that Brett was diagnosed with manic-depression and narcissism and that they had a volatile relationship, coming to near blows on several occasions. Andy asked Brett to meet with me so that I could explain his plans to her and obtain her agreement. Brett said she did not agree with Andy's approach to dementia and that she would not be able to keep him at home once his function started to diminish.

"I simply am not cut out to be a caregiver," she said.

"That's OK," Andy said. "Just make sure you stop my care as I ask. I won't live a long life with dementia but rather allow it to take me naturally."

Brett laughed and said, "I certainly will not. That would stop any checks from coming in."

She presented this as a joke, but Andy's face twisted into a worried grimace. I cautioned Andy that Brett may not be the most suitable durable power of attorney because they did not agree on the approach to care. Andy told me early on that he wanted to move to assisted living to relieve the pressure between him and Brett and to be able to live his life but allow her to keep the house and a portion of his pension and health care benefits.

"I will not divorce her no matter what," Andy said. "And it would break her heart if I didn't have her as my durable power of attorney. She will honor my wishes when the time comes; she is just adjusting right now."

As Andy was preparing to move to assisted living, he required an operation. He recovered in a rehabilitation facility and thought he would move to assisted living from there. But Brett canceled the planned move to assisted living, stating it was far too expensive and that she would care for Andy at home. Andy then realized that Brett was not going to honor his wishes. He debated with me and a trusted care coordinator whether he should obtain a voluntary conservatorship to change his power of attorney and protect himself. Brett convinced him she would be there for him, drive him where he needed to go, and support his journey living with dementia. They went home together.

Andy's support system, the physicians, social workers, music and art therapists, soon received notice that Andy would no longer be seeing us. I did not hear from Andy afterward except through a friend of his who reported that Andy sent greetings but was confined to home because Brett felt going out with him was too much work. I next saw Andy when he was admitted to the hospital after a hip fracture five years later. His dementia had markedly progressed, and he was entering late stages of the disease. Brett had him admitted to a skilled nursing facility after this hospitalization. Her plans were to continue his care as long as medically possible, including the insertion of a feeding tube if necessary.

---

In a recent report by Marguerite DeLiema of 53 cases sampled from an elder abuse forensics center, "trusted others" who had exploited an elder were described as children (40%), grandchildren (8%), other relative (4%), neighbors (16%), longtime friend (4%) and roommates/tenants (12%), nonrelative caregiver (8%), romantic partners (4%), and non–"trusted other" (4%). Exploitation is described as misuse of the older person's bank account funds or credit card, inappropriate transfer of property, falsely promising returns on investments when no returns were intended to be provided, falsely promising to provide care in exchange for payment when no care was intended to be provided, misappropriation of income and assets to benefit the perpetrator at the expense of the older person, and altering the older person's will or trust without consent.

Sixty-eight percent of exploitation victims were widowed, and many lived with the exploiter (36%). Based on neuropsychological reports, 64 percent of those exploited were intentionally isolated by the perpetrator, and 20 percent suffered from mental health issues (for example, bipolar disorder, substance abuse, or gambling issues) or had an established criminal record. This study suggests that a strong and active network of individuals advocating for an older adult is the best-case scenario.

─────────────── **POINTS TO REMEMBER** ───────────────

▶ Care partnering, especially as the family member with dementia is reaching the end of life, is full of complex and mixed emotions. The emotional state of the care partner significantly impacts how the care situation is perceived. Acknowledging the emotions that accompany caregiving and working to build resilience assist in the long journey of care partnering with someone living with dementia.

▶ Many wonderful experiences and personal growth can accompany the ups and downs of caregiving.

▶ Many of the difficult emotions that accompany caring for an individual living with dementia may be managed when good self-care practices are in place—good nutrition, sleep, respite, practicing joy.

▶ The relationship between the individual with dementia and the caregiver before the diagnosis of dementia may cloud the new relationship and roles. Be wary of holding onto old emotions and grudges and, if necessary, concede that care is best delivered by another.

▶ Be on guard for signs and symptoms of depression. Seek counseling and support at the earliest indications that the burden of caregiving is too much. Take advantage of all the resources you need to sustain your own well-being so that you can successfully assist in the care of your family member.

▶ Abuse and exploitation are not uncommon in caregiving. Be aware that isolation increases the likelihood that abuse and exploitation will occur. A full and vibrant social network is vital for both the care partner and the individual living with dementia.

---------------------------  ACTION PLAN  ---------------------------

▶ Begin a ritual to bring joy or happiness into every day. Whether you begin each day with a song, spend time meditating, praying or exercising, sharing a cup of tea and a two-minute funny YouTube clip, or enjoying pictures of family or a beautiful scene.

▶ Begin a gratitude journal every night recording one important, expansive, or beautiful experience that resulted from partnering in care with your family member.

▶ Keep a record of self-care with a checklist, including two to five servings of fruits or vegetables per day, six to eight hours of sleep each night, time away from home at least once per week, and a stress-relieving activity every day.

▶ Honor your temperament. If you need time alone, hire or barter for someone to provide care while you get away. If you need some time to socialize, find a group to invite over or go somewhere with your family member to fill your need. If you need order, spend 15 minutes every day decluttering and clearing in a mindful practice so that you can relax in your home. If your temperament is not conducive to direct care, so that you become verbally or physically abusive, contact your physician's office or a local social worker to discuss options for relinquishing daily caregiving to another qualified individual.

▶ At the end of your gratitude journal, outline the symptoms of depression and rate yourself. Crying, irritability, insomnia, increase or decrease in appetite, loss of enjoyment in most activities, overwhelming feelings of guilt or worthlessness, a decrease in energy, difficulty getting moving, and thoughts of suicide should be inventoried. Contact your physician if a few of these symptoms are present for more than a week or two or at any time that suicide is contemplated.

▶ The final inventory that needs attending to is a social network. Are you seeing people, either in person or via Skype? Direct interactions are important to avoid isolation. Plan and schedule time to engage with someone outside the home at least three times per week.

────────────── ADDITIONAL READING AND RESOURCES ──────────────

▶ *Caring for a Loved One with Dementia*, by Marguerite Manteau-Rao

This book offers a mindfulness-based approach to reducing stress when caregiving for an individual living with dementia. It includes an overview of the scientific background for the use of mindfulness for stress reduction, suggestion, and meditations to develop a mindfulness practice, and the use of mindfulness in coping with grief, approaches to daily tasks, activities, and situations common when living with dementia.

▶ *Just One Thing: Developing a Buddha Brain One Simple Practice at a Time*, by Rick Hanson

This source book includes 51 simple mental strategies to enhance positive brain activity and emotions. There is evidence that what we focus on changes our brain and what the brain thinks changes us. The book offers tested simple (so that we can actually adopt and master them) strategies to enhance inner peace, well-being, and emotional resilience.

▶ *Loving Someone Who Has Dementia*, by Pauline Boss

This guidebook helps caregivers cope with the stress and grief that accompanies caring for someone with dementia. Boss, a psychotherapist specializing in caregivers dealing with ambiguous loss (for example, spouses of prisoners of war or missing in action, caregivers of those with traumatic brain injury or dementia), simply and directly explains the differences faced when a family member is either physically missing but not known to be dead or cognitively lost but physically present. The complexities of coping and grieving and strategies to lessen the unusual burden are described.

# Making Decisions for Others

In many diseases, when the end comes the individual with the disease makes choices about how to treat *or not treat* the condition. In cancer, some opt for life-sustaining treatment no matter how slim the odds of success or how caustic the therapy. Those with bad knees from osteoarthritis may opt for surgical repair and a long recovery, while others choose only physical therapy or limit their functioning. Family members with differing opinions may push and prod, but, ultimately, the person with the condition is able to make his or her own choice. Not so with dementia. The disease renders the patient either literally or at least figuratively mute. As more decisions need to be made, identifying a surrogate decision maker or an appropriate other to make decisions is essential.

---

## MAKING ON-THE-SPOT DECISIONS
### • The Kenny Family Story •

It was my birthday. I had taken the day off and lay in bed, quietly thinking about some birthday wishes—some trivial about dinner plans and some more serious, that my mother would soon pass away peacefully. Minutes later, as if my wishes were somehow known, the phone rang. My mother was having trouble breathing; could they send her to the hospital? I was at her bedside within minutes and decided, no, she would not go to the hospital. Instead, we would call hospice to help control her symptoms of shortness of breath. This one occurrence held dozens of decisions and consequences. It was so difficult to see my mother working to breathe, groggy, struggling. But I also could imagine the scene if she went off to the hospital; the flurry of activity that she would not understand, the needles and oxygen masks, the new medications and their unknown effects in her delicate state.

---

Decisions, large and small, fall to caregivers or care partners. They run the gamut from deciding whether to struggle to shower someone who is vehemently resisting or to use antibiotics for the third episode of pneumonia. When you've become exhausted, can you afford to bring a paid caregiver into the home, or must you move your loved one to a skilled nursing facility? Is hospitalization the best choice, or should you do as much as you can to avoid a transfer to acute care? The list is endless. We may find ourselves alone making these tough, often overwhelming and frightening, decisions. In some cases, the decisions can or must be shared with others, such as a parent, a sibling or siblings, or a spouse. Then the intense emotions linked to these decisions may bump up against others so that the emotions take the front seat, more so than the decision.

Once the choices are made, we may need to defend them or advocate for them. My mother stayed home from the hospital; the caregivers at her dementia-specific assisted living were furious with me, feeling I was giving up on my mother. They felt that many families abandoned their charges to the care of strangers. If I hadn't had 25 years of watching patients hospitalized for limited benefit and seeing the potential for increased harm, I think the pressure from the facility caregivers would have altered my decisions. My family backed me, but I heard the uncertainty in their voices as they asked whether I was sure hospice was needed and how had our mother developed this shortness of breath so quickly?

We need to learn to build support for decision making for another—the support that will be needed to make and live well and comfortably with our decision.

# PRINCIPLES OF MAKING DECISIONS FOR OTHERS

Several ethical arguments provide the backbone for how medical decisions are valued. Much thought, theory, and legal battle have gone into many of these approaches, resulting in guidelines that, while fluid, do stand to help us understand what voice to bring to the table and what voice to favor.

Two of the basic human rights we value as a society are individual well-being and respect for individual self-determination. Individual well-being suggests that health and safety are components of well-being, but not the complete picture, so that only an individual can judge his or her own well-being. Physicians and health care providers may bring medical information and recommendations, but a person should weigh the risks and benefits to his or her entire life when making many of these medical decisions focused on well-being.

Going hand-in-hand with the principle of individual well-being is individual self-determination. Individuals may want input and guidance from others, but most prefer the ability to decide for themselves, to be in charge of their own lives. The two principles may conflict, when someone may make decisions (self-determination) that are not in the best interest of their own well-being. As a society, we must be careful of two scenarios—when we strip others of their ability to decide when they can make this decision and when we do not assist someone who is not able to make a decision. Evidence regarding a person's competence to make decisions is complex, decision specific, and often uncertain and conflicting. Unfortunately, therefore, there are no clear-cut procedures and standards to wash away or eliminate error in assisting with decision making. So we are left to wrestle with standards of competence. When an individual is in the late stages of dementia, competence to make medical decisions has nearly universally passed. To follow is the ethical framework or guidance principles that are often used to assist in surrogate decision making or decision making for another, once that decision has been made (see chapter 4, "Legal Aspects of Decisions"). The guidance principles are to make decisions that (a) promote the good of the individual (best interest), (b) accord with what the individual would decide if they could (substituted judgment), and (c) implement a declaration of advance directives made while the individual was deemed competent.

Because discrepancies may arise among the answers to the three guidance principles, the American Medical Association Code of Ethics orders the principles in situations in which more than one could be applied: For example, if a clear advance directive is valid, it takes precedence over best interest and substituted judgment. Documented advance directives allow individuals to retain control over health care decisions in anticipated situations and in unforeseen situations by choosing a trusted other to make decisions in their stead. It follows then to extend the individual's autonomy; if an individual does not have documented treatment preferences, the surrogate is asked to make decisions based on the patient preferences, taking into account previous discussions and values. The success of substituted judgment falls on the surrogate's ability to predict and honor the patient's preferences.

---

## LEARNING TO HONOR THE DECISIONS OF OTHERS
### • Mimi and Mildred's Story •

I was asked to speak with Mimi, the surrogate decision maker for her mother, Mildred, because of the frustration of the nursing staff. Mildred was living in a long-term care facility. She'd moved in 10 years ago when her decision-making capacity was good. She did well while attending the day program but was becoming anxious and frightened at night. She was close to Mimi but did not want to live with her or with an aide in her home. Mildred moved into skilled care, continuing to participate in the day program for several years, finding joy and meaning in socializing and assisting the nurses and aides. She had long chats with the nurses and Mimi about dementia and its progression during the evenings. She told all of them that she would like her final years to be peaceful. She did not want to be "carted" back and forth to the hospital with every infection or problem.

"It just tears these people up," Mildred said. "Something happens and they never come back themselves. We see it over and over. No . . . not for me. Once this disease has me that good, it is time to choose peace and quiet."

Mildred had reached that stage of dementia. She was suffering from repeated bouts of pneumonia, and Mimi kept having her go to the hospital. I sat with Mimi and Jean, the head nurse, to discuss the plan of care. After Jean reviewed with us how Mildred was functioning, I asked Mimi to tell me what she understood.

"Mom is at the end of her dementia and no longer knows me. She sleeps so much, but smiles so big when she's awake. She's getting pneumonia from eating, but with just a few days at the hospital, she comes right back here."

I asked what it is like for Mildred when she is in the hospital.

"Pure hell. She is scared and squirming all the time. They have to tie her down. But it's what we have to do to get her back here."

I said there are options other than going to the hospital. Mimi teared up immediately and said, "Not if I want her alive." I knew the answer before I asked because Jean had previously reported, but I asked Mimi what was most important to her mother. "Peace," she stated quietly. And to you? "Life," said Mimi. We sat in silence. "But I'm choosing for her—right?" "Yes," I said, "you're choosing for her." Mimi said, "I see, but it is so hard."

Jean hugged Mimi and said, "We'll help *you* with hard and help *your mom* with peace."

---

Mimi's story illustrates what can happen when the individual's and the surrogate's choices don't align. Fortunately, Mimi realized that her own wishes were tangled and interfering with Mildred's wishes. She needed time and support to come to the realization.

What happens when alignment doesn't occur? At times, making a decision requires obtaining input from an impartial third party. Ethics committees of institutions, such as hospitals or nursing homes, are often the first choice. The American Medical Association Principles of Medical Ethics suggests the following:

> Consult an ethics committee or other institutional resource when: (i) no surrogate is available or there is ongoing disagreement about who is the appropriate surrogate; (ii) ongoing disagreement about a treatment decision cannot be resolved; or (iii) the physician judges that the surrogate's decision: a. is clearly not what the patient would have decided when the patient's preferences are known or can be inferred; b. could not reasonably be judged to be in the patient's best interest; or c. primarily serves the interests of the surrogate or other third party rather than the patient. (AMA Principles of Medical Ethics: I, III, VIII)

When there is no direction for how an individual might decide on his or her care, the final principle is to base decisions on what would be in the person's best interest or would likely promote the greatest well-being. Many of the families I work with, initially, interpret this to mean choosing to prolong life. After questioning and discussing, families understand that well-being is broader than a simple life or death split. While there is no consensus on the definition of well-being, it is generally agreed to include the presence of positive moods and emotion, the absence of negative emotions, satisfaction with life, feelings of fulfillment and function. Although this list was created for academic investigation to understand and measure well-being, it can aid us in broadening our perspective to allow for decision making on behalf of someone else.

# BEING A SOLE DECISION MAKER

## BEING ALONE IN MAKING DECISIONS
## AND HAVING A BACKUP PLAN
### • *Carrie and James' Story* •

Carrie sat quietly in the corner, steam coming from her tea. A professional woman, she rose in rank faster than most in her field, taking on more and more responsibility and feeling the pressure from being a "first" or a "star." She credits her father, James, for role-modeling drive, leadership, and determination. Now, James is rapidly failing because of dementia, no longer able to drive or to live independently. His independent streak has made giving up decision making to Carrie difficult. Carrie asked to meet and discuss what to do because becoming the decision maker has left her feeling overwhelmed.

We chatted about her struggle to balance preserving her father's usual cogent decision making with overriding decisions that lacked his usual foresight and judgment. James's decline has necessitated that Carrie assume responsibility for daily decisions, and she was feeling the strain. "I can't believe how many details need to be attended to. His finances, medications, insurance questions, finding home health aides, begging and pleading after he fires home health aides, looking at alternative living options since he's walking away from the home health aides and beginning to fall. Everyone calls me. I'm interrupted at work, and I never make it home to the kids because I'm calming him down every night from the drama in the day. I know I'm lucky because we can afford some help but not for much longer. We can't keep the aides, his walking is worsening, and he'll need help to be lifted soon. It is time for Dad to move, but he doesn't want to. It feels like this is all coming to a head because I'm presenting at an international conference and will be gone for 10 days."

I asked whether Carrie had anyone supporting her during all these decisions and changes. "Ted, my husband, is great about

handling the kids, but I don't burden him with the details of Dad."
I then asked, "Is there anyone who can help you, to share the stress
with, or even if just to bounce off ideas? Do you have a backup plan
for your travels or when you go away?" Carrie placed her head in
her hands and sighed deeply.

---

Some family members are grateful to be able to make decisions
as a surrogate and may even prefer to be the sole decision maker.
Being the sole decision maker eliminates concerns about accurate
communication and understanding about goals and plans that may
occur with multiple decision makers. However, being the sole decision maker also comes with burdens, including the scope, intensity,
and duration of the responsibility.

## THE SCOPE OF AND PREPARATION FOR THE RESPONSIBILITY IN CAREGIVING

The scope of the responsibility for care is broad. In Carrie and James's
situation, Carrie was concerned about finances, medications, safety,
her father's quality of life and autonomy, insurance, and housing.
Caregivers are often responsible for not only physical care but also
medication administration and assessing for side effects, with limited
or no medical knowledge—a very stressful situation. Carol Levine,
director of the Families and Health Care Project for the United Hospital Fund of New York, writes in the executive summary of *Rough
Crossings: Family Caregivers' Odysseys through the Health Care System*
that caregivers are usually thrust into their role by necessity, though
most want to provide the care because the person was significant in
their lives. It is this tender concern for the family member that further leads to anxiety and fear for the family member's welfare. The
intensity of the responsibility extends from this lack of preparation.
Much of the skills for caregiving are self-taught, found by searching

the Internet or calling on friends with health care experience. Transitions from hospitals and from periods of home health coverage do offer education, but family caregivers feel the preparation is brief and inadequate. Finally, the duration of care and decision making is prolonged, causing fatigue and burnout.

Further responsibilities for financial, insurance, and housing needs are also complicated by the limited preparation. Understanding community resources and how to access them when needed is frequently not known or well communicated by health care providers to family members. Interventions that have provided education and communication about available community resources have demonstrated reduced stress and improved quality of life for caregivers. Delegating and using available resources assist the caregiver, especially one who is a sole decision maker, in decreasing stress and developing a network and backup plan to provide adequate care for a family member.

## THE IMPORTANCE OF A BACKUP PLAN
## FOR CAREGIVING

What about the importance of a backup plan? Times of travel or sickness are inevitable, and the surrogate decision maker should be prepared. Most times, when a durable power of attorney is selected, a successor is also named. Communication with the successor should be ongoing so that transition of responsibility is seamless in an acute situation. Times of travel may be an excellent time to update communication. If no successor is available, the durable power of attorney should secure someone to fill this role. Reasonable choices would be a family member or close friend who feels comfortable stepping in. If no one is available, geriatric care managers, lawyers, and social workers are reliable and guided by codes of ethics to serve as conservator. Assistance can be found on the Alzheimer's Association community resource finder at http://www.communityresourcefinder.org/.

## SHARING DECISION MAKING

Making end-of-life decisions can be complex and stir many issues, concerns, and triggers in each of us. When we need to include several people in the decisions being made for another person, some sticky, layered conversations may be unearthed. What is the best way to begin? Try beginning with yourself and ask yourself questions about your values, beliefs, wishes, and fears for your end of life. Take some time, space, and solitude to imagine this. Maybe you could take a quiet walk in the woods, a warm bath, or go for a peaceful car ride. Using a checklist may help you hit some highlights. See Table 3.1 for suggested questions. Once you've done this for yourself, take a bit of time to consider your family member—does he or she share your perspective? Come to the same conclusions? What questions would you need to ask health care professionals, legal experts, social workers, or religious leaders to understand options for your scenarios? What life stories from your family member would assist you in answering these questions in his or her place? It would be helpful for each of the shared decision makers to go through a similar exercise, considering themselves to truly feel the depth of the question (and create a document for their surrogate decision makers) and assist them in coming to some conclusions for their family member.

It is then time to come together to make decisions. Some families do this proactively. My mother had the forethought to do this for us. Each of her children had varied expertise in law, finance, medicine, communication, and spiritual matters. She delegated responsibilities to each of us early so that we understood where we each needed to provide input as part of the family. She delegated several of us as durable power of attorney to act on her behalf as her cognitive abilities deteriorated. We may not have always agreed on all aspects of her care, but we were respectful of our mother's wishes for peace, civility, and expertise. We, as a family, kept our mother's goals and wishes center to our decisions. I know this is not always the way things progress for every family, but it is a worthwhile goal to work toward.

**TABLE 3.1** End-of-Life Review to Assist with Decision Making

| CONCEPT | QUESTIONS | WHO MIGHT ASSIST |
| --- | --- | --- |
| Values | Do you have a vision for how you'd want to die? | Family |
| | Who would be with you? | Friends |
| | Where would you be? | |
| | What are the limits you'd live with as a guide to those who may need to make decisions for you? | |
| | Are there things you'd like to accomplish before your death? | |
| Legacy | Do you have a legacy? | Family |
| | Financial, stories, treasures? | Friends |
| | How and to whom do you want to pass this along? | |
| Physical | Are there limitations you do not feel you could tolerate? | Family |
| | What physical risks are you willing to tolerate to live alone? Ability to walk? Have privacy? Or is safety your top concern? | Friends |
| | | Health care providers |
| Emotional | What emotional state is important? | Family |
| | What sacrifices would you withstand to keep this? | Friends |
| | | Counselors |
| | Have you addressed issues that burden you, for example, limiting beliefs, addictions, regrets? | Spiritual leaders |
| Spiritual | Are you satisfied with your spiritual affairs? | Family |
| | Are you comfortable with making amends, working on forgiveness of yourself and others, surrendering negative self-talk, compassion? | Friends |
| | | Spiritual leaders |
| | | Counselors |

**TABLE 3.1** *(continued)*

| CONCEPT | QUESTIONS | WHO MIGHT ASSIST |
|---|---|---|
| Financial | How important is fiscal prudence in your decisions? | Lawyers<br>Financial advisers |
| | What level of financial burden would you tolerate to accomplish your goals? | |
| | Do you have your financial affairs in order, including wills, long-term care insurance, life insurance, funeral plans? | |

## END-OF-LIFE STRESS MAY UNMASK FAMILY STRIFE

Often, the time of death or decline of the patriarch or matriarch of a family brings about poor communication and strife. Defense mechanisms of denial, repressed feelings, projection, bullying, and anger may surface. I have seen many families with deep disagreements, digging in their heels in what appears to be impassable conflict. When the level of trust in a family is low, the time of end-of-life decisions adds an overwhelming layer of stress that heightens the discourse. And most families are somewhere between the extremes of my family, with my mother's forethought and cooperative siblings, and the deeply entrenched, distrustful family. So what is a way forward when there is discord?

## SAFE COMMUNICATION IS KEY

Several books are available on communication, especially in difficult times. I highly recommend *Crucial Conversations* by Patterson, Grenny, McMillan, and Switzler. In this book, crucial conversations are defined as those between individuals when stakes are high, opinions vary, and emotions run strong. The authors give advice, experience, and examples of leading with your heart and focusing on what your goals are, not on your reaction or defense to opinions or attacks from others. The book coaches to observe for times when feelings of safety are breached so that you can be aware of where the conversation can go awry, especially through withdrawing from communication or verbally attacking rather than communicating. Because having conversations about end-of-life issues for a family member are required, strategies and exercises on how to make the conversations safe for all parties involved are covered. The authors outline common narratives we tell ourselves to rationalize why conversations cannot occur and provide strategies for moving beyond these impasses. Finally, the authors also include strategies on how to make decisions when there is not a clear authority on a decision, as may occur in shared surrogate decision making.

Several questions help to decide how to proceed in a clear fashion: Who cares or genuinely wants to be involved in the decision making? Who has expertise to assist in the decision? Who must agree or cooperate to make the decision, and how many people need to be involved? With answers to these questions, you can decide whether to obtain expertise from outside your group and whether decisions will be made by one or all. I've seen families vote, but I highly recommend the group comes to consensus. Although all may not agree with all aspects of the decision, all should agree that the family member for whom decisions are being made would choose this. If even one member of the group disagrees, I recommend waiting on final decisions, because usually a common ground can be found if that individual is given some time and a voice.

---

### DISAGREEING WITH OTHERS TO THE POINT OF BROKEN RELATIONSHIPS

#### • *The Whites' Story* •

We met in a large conference room to discuss the mixed and confusing recommendations the Whites were receiving on their father's medical course and whether he was at the point of death. The family resemblance among the three sisters was such that they appeared to be triplets, but their body language lacked any warmth or compassion for one another. They each sat stiffly and positioned their bodies to exclude one sister, Brianna, the power of attorney and decision maker. She had worked hard to understand all her father's medical complications and to please her sisters' need for control and information. Her sisters refused to budge on cooperating with her or the health care team that had convened to assist them.

The health care team asked questions to understand about their father and his history, wants, and desires. Bethany and Brooke sat rigidly, addressing each question by stating what they wanted or by attacking the decisions Brianna had made thus far. In response, Brianna would bristle and jump in to defend herself. Brianna's husband, Bob, would lay his hand across her arm trying to calm her and keep her from reacting. The sisters were entangled in a deep tug-of-war. After some time of laying the groundwork, with each sister stating how she felt and the health care team confirming their individual feelings, the conversation seemed to move forward to a place where a plan of action might be possible. But each sister had laid traps for the others, so no matter the outcome with their father, unresolved resentment and anger would persist. We attempted to discuss that this may be a time for healing and support, but there was no sense of safety in the conversation. These sisters were about to lose their father to death and their family to anger. The level of sadness in the room was profound.

---

Another excellent resource for communicating effectively is Marshall B. Rosenberg's *Nonviolent Communication*. The strategies outlined in this book would help the White family find a way toward peace and connection. One of my goals in working with many families is to help them make decisions together and maintain a strong family unit, even when all do not agree. Many families do not need the more in-depth insights of *Nonviolent Communication* and can come to agreements using skills reviewed in *Crucial Conversations*, but for families with more complex relationships and deep underlying communication issues, the exercises and insights from *Nonviolent Communication* can provide guidance to allow for understanding and compassion. Nonviolent communication involves language and communication skills that strengthen our ability to tap into our humanness, even under stressful or difficult conditions. The practice is consciously expressing ourselves and hearing others from a place of honesty, clarity, and compassion, rather than automatic reactions. The skills built when using nonviolent communication break patterns of defending, withdrawing, or attacking in the face of judgment and criticism. The goals of all interactions then focus on communication while maintaining the relationship.

Rosenberg reviews that it is a societal norm to learn communication styles that are alienating to others, such as judgments, comparisons, and demands. He recommends building the skill of observing and reporting without evaluation. Evaluation is seen as criticism and shuts down communication. He then recommends expressing how we feel—a skill most of us have not mastered. Recently, I found myself feeling frustrated, angry, and negative about the hopes of my child competing successfully for admittance to a graduate program. But when I checked in on these quick and deep negative emotions, I realized I just hadn't let myself feel sadness watching my son struggle with the process and uncertainty of acceptance to the program. Once I clearly felt the sadness, I was open to supporting my son, rather than to feeling judgment or anger.

When feelings can be identified, nonviolent communication encourages making requests that enrich life, rather than requests that "win" or "acquiesce." Brianna displayed deep sadness and depression as she tried to mold her actions to please her sisters, who used vague language that allowed for chastising Brianna no matter what she said. If Brianna had been true to herself and able to ask her sisters to consider concrete actions, such as "I would like you to acknowledge that I gathered medical information from five physicians to review so that we could all be informed and discuss this together," that may have allowed enough of an opening for the women to see they had some common ground. If the listener is able to meet the request, the step should be acknowledged, a gesture that keeps the conversation moving in a give-and-take way. The request cannot be seen as a demand, or the system breaks down.

Empathy, compassion, and self-compassion are required for the strategies in *Nonviolent Communication* to enhance communication. The book outlines how to listen empathetically with presence, paraphrasing, focusing on feelings rather than logic, and consciously exploring what need is fulfilled with each choice (for example, money, approval, shame, sense of duty).

## REACTIONS FROM OTHERS REGARDING DECISIONS

### STANDING UP TO OTHERS WHO DISAGREE
#### • *Carmen's Story* •

Carmen was sitting slouched in a chair with her feet on her mother's wheelchair. Her mother, Rosa, was asleep in the specialized chair, tipped into a reclined position so her head was well supported. Carmen smiled at me as I approached, but her expression changed to one of sadness and worry as she looked at her mother. Carmen, only in her mid-20s, had recently petitioned the court to become conservator for her mother, rather than a lawyer. Carmen reported that she'd been making many of the decisions for her mother for years but had been too young to do it legally.

"There is so much disagreement in my family on what is best for Mom, so the courts got involved. But I know she is at the end of her life, and we need to leave her in peace. My uncles called me 'devil child' and worse when I insisted she move into a facility. But she has taken off on me several times—how was I supposed to take care of her if she wouldn't even stay in the house?" Carmen continued to talk about her difficulties with family, compounded because her mother was so young when diagnosed with dementia. "They all think there is something that can be done to turn this around, especially my uncles. They tell me to make the facility find a way to get her to eat or wake her up or make her walk. No one but me has the . . . courage . . . to see that this can't be stopped. And no one but me has the courage to make the difficult decisions."

---

Carmen illustrates that it can be difficult on the decision maker, who takes the time and energy to understand the disease and the inevitability of its progression. Carmen found the personal strength to stand up to family when she was attacked for her decisions. She found an ally in a brother, which she said helps. He won't make the decisions, but he will back her up with other family members. She said this is enough for her. I worked with a therapist to help deal with my feelings of strain when I was confronted with resistance from facility caregivers in the decisions I made for my mother. Several of the families I've worked with have found backing from friends and clergy. Others have found only those in a support group can understand the complexities of making life-and-death decisions for someone else in the face of disagreement.

## HELPFUL STRATEGIES TO SUPPORT THE DECISION MAKER

What is reported to help a decision maker in times of stress? Sometimes language or examples of ways to discuss your decisions can be helpful. My colleague uses a definitive but gracious response when she is asked to join a committee or pile on another task to her already overburdened schedule: "I couldn't possibly." Are there ways like this to counter someone who challenges a decision? When someone said, "I could never put my mother in a home" or "How can you [fill in the blank] (for example, stop medications, start hospice, move him to a home, go on vacation when she lingers)?" I found a good response was something to the effect of "All of these decisions are so complex. For my mother and family, we've carefully considered so many options and feel comfortable this is the best solution for us." The statement was positive and affirming and showed that a team of people had input, including my mother. There were no apologies or pleading or defending. My family's decisions were well thought out and the best in our situation—a situation that I felt did not need to be seen as either good or bad.

Dealing with criticism may not be pleasant but it is easier to do if you are confident in your decisions and have good self-esteem. Unfortunately, the stress of caregiving may require these decisions to be made when you are tired, have been neglecting self-care, and may feel underconfident. At times like this, criticism may leave you feeling hurt, angry, and confused. What are some strategies to deal with criticism when you are not sure of your decision? First, step back from any feelings of defensiveness. If you don't take the comments personally, you will have a better chance of exploring whether there is any truth in the criticism, which can serve as a natural check on your choice. If, when the criticism is evaluated from a less emotional, more objective stance, you feel that the information is accurate, that there is no misunderstanding and that the critic is not trying to deliberately hurt you, you can thank the critic for his or her insight and move on to gather more information if needed and take some additional time to consider all options. You may well stick with your original decision, but you've now had time to calm down and should now be more confident that you've truly explored any additional options.

---
### POINTS TO REMEMBER

▸ Decisions about day-to-day needs and the end-of-life process are left to the care partners of those with dementia because the disease has rendered the individual unable to speak for himself or herself.

▸ The ethical framework for surrogate decision making includes individual well-being and respect for individual self-determination.

Guidance from the idea of promoting the good of the individual then follows, making decisions according to their wishes and implementing any prestated declaration of advance care planning.

▶ When there is no one to make decisions or there are ongoing disagreements with decisions, institutional ethics committees can assist in resolving conflict.

▶ Education and seeking counsel from others enmeshed in end-of-life decisions (for example, spiritual counselors, lawyers, social workers, hospice workers) can be helpful to individuals and groups faced with making choices for another.

▶ Shared decision making can unearth or heighten strained relationships and communication among family members. The use of established, researched, and tested strategies may be helpful in navigating communication or hiring a mediator when needed to facilitate the thorniest discussions.

▶ When surrogates are faced with criticism for decisions they've made, information and distance from intense emotions can help in coming to a confident decision that can be communicated to others, even when they may not agree.

──────────────────── ACTION PLAN ────────────────────

▶ Use Table 3.1 to review your own thoughts about how you want to consider end-of-life issues. Once you've explored your own thoughts and opinions, imagine yourself in your family member's shoes and readdress the issues from his or her perspective and journey with dementia. If you are making decisions with others, ask them to participate in the same exercise to prepare for a group discussion.

▶ If you are making decisions alone for a family member, consider who would make decisions in your stead (in case of emergency) and ask and advise that individual immediately of information and rights needed in that scenario.

▶ Acquaint yourself with principles of surrogate decision making such as substituted judgment and promoting the good of the individual.

▶ Develop a network and keep a list of trusted "others" that can be used for counsel during times of difficult decisions—clergy, spiritual counselors, social workers, community resources (many towns have experts in social services to assist with understanding resources, lawyers, geriatric case managers). You can meet people such as these at support groups, local area talks, your Area Agency on Aging, or through your physician's office.

▶ Work on communication skills using resources recommended or with a therapist to enhance your decision-making capabilities and maintain your sense of confidence in this difficult time.

―――――――――    **ADDITIONAL READING AND RESOURCES**    ―――――――――

▶ *Crucial Conversations*, by Kerry Patterson, Joseph Grenny, Ron McMillan, and Al Switzler

This book, filled with stories, exercises, and examples, assists the reader in understanding the importance of engaging in difficult conversations. The authors highlight common defensive actions that deflect good communication. The authors give a good overview on how to logically sort through who may be the best decision maker when there is uncertainty on authority in decisions.

▶ *Nonviolent Communication*, by Marshall B. Rosenberg

Dr. Rosenberg, a psychotherapist and educator/innovator in nonviolent communication, describes the steps to improve effective, compassionate, and heartfelt communication. There are strategies for conflict resolution and mediation. The theories and practices from this book are often used or recommended by institutions to coach those with anger management and poor interpersonal relationships. Workshops are sponsored internationally and endorsed by the Center for Nonviolent Communication (www.CNVC.org).

# Legal Aspects of Decisions

So many families are caught off guard by the legal aspects of decision making. Without legal planning and preparation, maneuvering the health care, financial, and business needs of a family member is extremely difficult. If no one has been designated a durable power of attorney, health care professionals will address the next of kin, who may or may not be the most reasonable or reliable individual to take on decisions.

This chapter will review the common legal situations faced by those with end-stage dementia and their families and caregivers, including issues of decision making, common insurance situations, and estate dissolution. A financial and legal plan is important and hopefully has been addressed in the earliest stage of dementia. Several guides are available to assist in both understanding legal documents that are needed or desired and finding an attorney who specializes in assistance to those living with dementia. Because state laws differ, it is crucial to check any general comments with someone who is knowledgeable about the laws in your state.

---

### HAVING LEGAL DOCUMENTS IN PLACE
#### • *The Kenny Family Story* •

We sat in the lawyer's office. My mother had spoken with my brother, an accountant, and asked how she could ensure that she and her second husband would not financially wipe out the other if one of them needed nursing home care. Thankfully, she had started this conversation early in her dementia, a testament to her frugality and practicality. If she had not, we would not have begun the process of setting her legal affairs in order. We would not have established her durable power of attorney, would not have discussed long-term care insurance policies, would not have talked about her wishes if she would become unable to make decisions for herself. We were lucky. Almost immediately after the visit to the lawyer, my mother's life took a drastic turn when her husband became acutely ill and required skilled nursing care, and her ability to live on her own was lost. Having these legal documents in place eased the multiple transitions that followed: selling her home, moving to assisted living, securing supplemental care, and so forth. Without these documents in place, we would have entered the undesirable legal world of guardianship and capacity.

---

## LEGAL PLANNING

Legal and financial issues are certainly best dealt with earlier rather than later in the course of dementia, but many of us only start to become involved later in the disease process. For that reason, definitions and overviews of common questions are reviewed in this chapter. The key to making legal and financial decisions rests in values, about life and your hopes, dreams, and fears about the end stage of your disease. These conversations can be difficult, but I have found that most people are relieved to be asked and have an opportunity to share. Death and dying are often considered taboo subjects, but once the conversation has been broached, meaningful and touching conversations can ensue.

When my mother was first diagnosed, I visited her and invited her to engage in an intimate conversation. I made sure my kids were being cared for, that the conversation was in the middle of the day so we were both rested, and that we had a private, comfortable place to talk. I started by bringing up my father's sudden death and how it was such a shock to us all. I apologized for being so blunt but asked my mom if she had thought about her own death. I told her I wanted to respect her wishes and make sure events unfolded the way she wanted them to. She had chosen me as her health care proxy, and I wanted to make sure I knew how best to make decisions if and when she couldn't any longer. She admitted she had been thinking about it since she had been diagnosed with dementia. After my father's death, she had trained as a clown and volunteered in long-term care facilities. She talked about the individuals she met who could no longer speak, walk, or care for themselves and how many had seemed so unhappy. We used this experience as a springboard to discuss options for what could and, conversely, didn't have to be done. We talked about hospice. We talked about types of living options and her financial situation that would support those options. We reconfirmed who she wanted to make decisions for her when she could no longer make her own—she designated legal, financial, and medical decisions to different individuals. She had long ago made decisions about resuscitation and intubation, but we talked about whether there were other medical situations that she found unsettling or fear inducing and for which she might want to make a decision in advance.

When these types of questions are first brought up, many of my patients, unlike my mother, are not ready to have a discussion. I ask them to think things through and come back, possibly with family members to talk. It is a good idea for family care partners to be present so that two or more family members hear my request. I even suggest that this task is their "homework," and I highly recommend using the Conversation Project Starter Kit (http://theconversation project.org/starter-kits/), from the Institute for Healthcare Improvement, founded by Ellen Goodman and Len Fishman. The homework provides the momentum and the tool kit provides the process to begin bringing the taboo subject of medical and legal decisions into a more open discussion. The Conversation Project Starter Kit focuses on values and wishes to guide those who may need some help making end-of-life decisions.

What if dementia has progressed to the point that your family member can no longer make their wishes clear? Chapter 3, "Making Decisions for Others," discusses the principles that should be considered in this circumstance. The most important point is to ask yourself how your family member would answer such important end-of-life questions. Did your family member ever discuss the health and life of others that would provide clues to what he or she would want? Were there discussions of movies or books or celebrity lives that informed your impression of your family member's opinions of care options at the end of life?

*Competency/Capacity: Competency* has a legal definition referring to an individual's ability to make decisions. It is a broad concept encompassing many legally recognized activities, such as the ability to enter into a contract, to prepare a will, to stand trial, and to make medical decisions. It is decided by the courts, and individuals are presumed to be competent unless proven otherwise. *Capacity*, however, refers to an assessment of the individual's psychological abilities to form rational decisions, specifically the individual's ability to understand, appreciate, and manipulate information and form rational decisions. Physicians, therefore, often make decisions on someone's capacity to make reasoned medical decisions, and if an individual's capacity is found lacking, then others are relied on to assist in decision making. This is referred to as de facto incompetent, that is, incompetent in fact but not determined to be so by legal procedures. Capacity is not always clear in all individuals, especially those living with dementia. One may be able to make some but not all medical decisions in earlier stages of the disease, depending on what areas of cognition and executive function—the set of mental skills that allow us to organize activities, pay attention, and get things done—are affected. In the last stages of dementia, an individual is thought to lack capacity for decisions regarding medical care and require a surrogate decision maker such as a power of attorney, health care proxy, or guardian.

*Durable Power of Attorney / Durable Power of Attorney for Health Care:* A durable power of attorney for health care is a document that lets you name someone else to make decisions about your health care in case you are not able to make those decisions yourself. It gives that person (called your agent) instructions about the kinds of medical treatment you want (and don't want) to ensure that your wishes are honored even if you are physically or mentally unable to communicate them. If you have not decided or declared your specific wishes, you should choose someone you trust to make the decisions in your stead. The durable power of attorney must be in writing; the person named must be over 18 years old and does not have to be a family member. More than one durable power of attorney for health care may be chosen, either coagents so that they share equal rights to make decisions or successively so that one has primary rights and if not available, the other can act in the primary agent's place. Agents are not required to act by law, but if they do act, they must follow your wishes (if you've stated them in writing or in person).

If you have not declared a durable power of attorney for health care and are physically or mentally unable to communicate your health care wishes, the following people, in order of priority, are legally authorized to make your health care decisions for you: court-appointed guardian or conservator, spouse or domestic partner, an adult child, an adult sibling, a close friend, or a nearest living relative. In the medical system, this usually works out, but it can cause stress and quarrels when family members do not agree. The durable power of attorney for health care assists in mitigating these quarrels.

Your agent can make a wide range of health care decisions, including whether to admit or discharge you from a hospital or nursing home, which treatments or medicines to receive, and who has access to your medical records. Your agent is not liable for making decisions for you as long as he or she is acting "in good faith" and/or following your direction.

In addition to the durable power of attorney for health care, an individual can designate a financial or general power of attorney, which authorizes someone to make decisions in financial or other matters. There can be both a durable power of attorney for health care and a durable financial or general power of attorney. The individuals chosen for the agents can be the same or different people.

The durable power of attorney for health care, finances, or general must be chosen and formally named via a written document when the individual naming them is cognitively able to make the decision. The agents may be revoked and another chosen, but again, this must be done when the individual is cognitively able to make the decision. It is important to know that a general power of attorney agent's power ends if the grantor becomes mentally incapacitated, necessitating the use of a durable power of attorney, which remains in effect even in the case of mental incapacity.

A lawyer is not required to establish a durable power of attorney but should probably be consulted if you plan to establish one. There are nuances that should be considered about what authorities you will relinquish and when.

*Guardianship/Conservator:* A guardian is a person, institute, or agency appointed by a court to manage someone's personal affairs, such as finances, housing, and medical decisions. The term *conservator* is sometimes used rather than guardian, or sometimes conservator is used solely for the financial aspects of another's affairs. It is possible to have both a guardian to make personal, nonmonetary decisions and a conservator to handle financial decisions, such as investments. Laws vary for different states, but generally, guardianship or conservatorship is sought when the individual living with dementia is deemed incapable of understanding or communicating decisions about personal or financial matters and a durable power of attorney was not selected before the loss of capacity.

Guardianship is a legal proceeding, such that one person (the petitioner) sues another individual (either the person with dementia or another guardian) for the legal right to make decisions for the person with dementia. The court will then assess several things: the appropriateness of the need for guardianship and the care plan for the individual. A medical and/or psychiatric evaluation is done to assess mental capacity of the individual to aid in the decision about appropriateness. In addition, the court will evaluate the current and/or potential guardian for management of the individual's affairs, including financial issues, medical decisions, and care needs.

The courts appoint the guardian to ensure the individual (for whom the legal term is *ward*) is well cared for and safe. The court usually appoints a close family member, but other relatives or friends can be considered. If there is no family or friend available, the court will appoint a neutral individual who is trained in handling guardianship matters, often a lawyer. Guardianship is usually reserved for situations in which disputes over opinions on proper care cannot be resolved. An example would be when an individual does not believe he or she has cognitive loss and refuses assistance. If the individual is becoming a threat to self or others, a family member may proceed with a request for guardianship. The court will appoint a guardian ad litem to assist the individual who has been served with papers to be an independent, objective advocate during the guardianship process. The guardian ad litem will obtain an attorney to represent the ward, and arrange for a mental examination and interpretation (usually performed by a physician). The guardian ad litem will gather information from the ward and family, friends, and interested parties and then report to the judge. The judge will then decide on need for guardianship and who will serve in that role.

Another example of when guardianship may be requested is when there is family disagreement on care or concerns for exploitation. The court may be petitioned to evaluate the appropriateness of one person over another to serve as guardian.

The proceedings for permanent guardianship are lengthy, often lasting several months to a year. Emergency guardianship may be requested if quick decisions are needed to avoid injury or risk of harm. Emergency guardianship is temporary and serves as a bridge until proceedings are conducted to determine permanent guardianship. Guardianship is a serious matter that intrudes on personal liberties and is therefore considered as a last resort when other alternatives have not been successful. Other forms of assistance such as living wills, trusts, case management, and powers of attorney are more common and preferred ways of providing appropriate assistance to someone who is living with dementia. If guardianship is granted by the court, the guardian is responsible for the ward and to report to the court on the ward and/or his or her estate on a regular basis.

*Advance Directives*: Advance directives are written instructions that provide information on your goals and wishes if you were seriously ill, dying, or living with a long-term chronic, disabling condition such as Alzheimer disease or related dementias. They are prepared when an individual has mental capacity. Your living will is a piece of advance directives, focused specifically on resuscitation, intubation, and feeding at the end of life. Because a living will is limited in scope, the use of a health care proxy or durable power of attorney is suggested. This person should be someone you trust to follow your wishes and directives. Information on how to establish a living will, a health care proxy, or a durable power of attorney (for health care or in general) can be found on state and local websites, at your physician's office, and from several private organizations promoting patients' rights (such as the Conversation Project, www.conversationproject .org). The forms usually require a witness and sometimes a notarized witness. Copies of your paperwork should be shared with your physician and your health care proxy and kept in your own files.

I recommend reviewing health care decisions on an annual basis. Some of my patients use their birthday, one uses tax day (getting all the messy stuff over at one time), and another schedules her review at the time of her yearly colonoscopy. The creativity of my patients never fails to keep me giggling; many people know how to take a serious task and give it some levity. The annual review is also a time to see if you believe your health care proxy continues to be a wise choice. Illness or other life circumstances may have intervened in their lives as well, changing their ability to help you. Finally, if you spend significant time in more than one area (e.g., traveling to see grandchildren or staying in an out-of-state vacation home), check to see that your living will and health care proxy documents are adequate for your second state or fill them out for that region.

*Physician Orders for Life Sustaining Treatment (POLST, also known as MOLST or POST):* The National POLST Paradigm is an approach to advance care planning developed for patients with one or more serious illnesses or frailty. It is for individuals whose life expectancy is approximately one year or less. It is written by a physician, after a conversation between the patient (or surrogate) and the health care professional. The POLST conversation is about the disease, treatment options and alternatives, and what the patient would want done based on his or her goals of care and values. After the conversation, the health care provider fills out a POLST form, marking what treatments can be chosen (or not chosen) at the end of your life. Because the POLST is a medical order, it means that your treatment wishes will be known and should be followed during a medical emergency (including by emergency medical system [EMS] personnel). The form is brightly colored and only one page. It is usually kept in an open area, such as tacked to the door of the bedroom, at the foot of the bed, or on the refrigerator door so that it is easy to locate. The movement is developing throughout the United States. It is developing, endorsed, or fully implemented in 45 of the 50 states thus far.

## FINANCIAL PLANNING

The largest proportion of a household budget often goes to housing and health care, and it is these two aspects that are likely to dramatically change for a person living with dementia. Unfortunately, we often don't plan for changes. Studies report that 70 percent of Americans older than 65 will need long-term care at some time, but most don't understand how it is structured or paid for. The need for long-term care tends to increase with advancing age, being a woman (because women generally outlive men), living alone, and having a chronic illness or illnesses that lead to some type of disability. The diagnosis of dementia puts someone at a high risk of requiring long-term care, because the disease is chronic but progressive and usually occurs in those with advanced age.

It is important to estimate your need for care and where you will likely need to be to receive that care to assist in financial planning. To assess these needs, consider who will provide care and in what setting it will be required. From these considerations and scenarios and information on current financial situation, thoughtful plans and options can be explored.

## INSURANCE OR PAYING FOR THE COST OF CARE

Dementia care can be expensive, both directly in costs of durable medical equipment, medications, and incontinence products, and indirectly in the time and expense of informal caregiving. As outlined in chapter 8, caregivers expend many dollars of personal expenses to care for someone living with dementia. It is therefore important to know what resources are available to you. Care is divided into medical care and personal care. Medical care is paid for via insurance.

*Medicare*: Medicare is the federal health insurance program for people who are 65 or older, certain younger people with disabilities, and people with end-stage renal disease (permanent kidney failure requiring dialysis or a transplant, sometimes called ESRD). Medicare Part A (hospital insurance) covers hospital stays, qualified skilled nursing and home health care, and hospice care. Medicare Part B covers certain physician and outpatient services, medical supplies, and preventive services such as immunizations. Medicare Part C (Medicare Advantage Plans) is a specific type of Medicare health plan provided by a private insurance company that contracts with Medicare for both Part A and Part B services. Each Part C plan has specific nuances and should be carefully reviewed for your specific circumstances. Medicare Part D (prescription drug coverage) is also offered by private insurance companies to add prescription drug coverage to the original Part A and Part B plans. Full information on Medicare can be found at www.medicare.gov.

Medicare coverage is based on federal and state laws. National coverage decisions are made by Medicare, and local coverage decisions are made by companies that process Medicare claims. The Medicare website has links to assist in exploring whether a test or service is covered. If it is not, you may be able to discuss with your physician or health care professional whether there is a real need or an alternative way to request the item or service.

Medicare doesn't cover all medical costs. For this reason, several individuals carry Medicare gap coverage. Gap coverage is important because of Medicare deductibles, coinsurance, and copayments. In addition, important services not covered by Medicare that should be considered in financial planning include long-term care (also called *custodial care*), dental care and dentures, eye examinations related to prescribing glasses, hearing aids and audiology exams for fitting hearing aids, routine foot care, cosmetic surgery, and acupuncture. Most important for those living with dementia, Medicare does not pay for nonskilled assistance with activities of daily living, such as dressing, bathing, and toileting, which make up the majority of needs.

## PRIVATE HEALTH INSURANCE

Medigap policies are often purchased privately to cover deductibles, copayments, or coinsurance not covered by the Medicare typical coverage. Medigap policies are provided by private insurance companies, require that you are enrolled in Medicare Part A and Part B, and carry a premium in addition to the premium for Medicare Part B.

Individuals may have private health insurance that is not a Medigap policy. Private health insurance may be provided by an employer or obtained through a union, or individuals may purchase coverage on their own. It is important to understand your policy's lifetime maximums or other limitations because dementia has a long period of disability, and coverage may not last for the duration of the disease. It is also important to continue payments, so as not to lose coverage. Because of the cognitive decline of my mother's spouse, he missed payments for his insurance, which resulted in long, burdensome, unsuccessful appeals by his daughters in an attempt to right the matter.

## LONG-TERM CARE

Long-term care refers to a set of services and supports for activities of daily living, such as dressing, bathing, eating, and moving around. Medicare and private insurance does not generally pay for long-term care. Medicaid (described in the next section) may assist in payment for long-term care but the conditions are specific.

Almost half of the formal long-term care provided in the United States is paid out of pocket. While not every person with Alzheimer disease needs long-term care, most do, and it is prudent to develop a plan due to the cost of long-term care.

Various ways to pay for long-term care include long-term care insurance, reverse mortgages, life insurance options, and annuities. Long-term care insurance eligibility is often limited, especially if certain medical conditions already exist, such as dementia. A reverse mortgage is a home equity loan that provides cash against the value of the house without selling the home. There are special rules to qualify for a reverse mortgage, including using the home as the primary residence (therefore providing resources to pay for in-home long-term care). Some life insurance policies have accelerated death benefits that allow a tax-free advance on the life insurance (though these extra benefits may require an extra premium). Finally, annuities can be purchased (for example, when you do not qualify for long-term care insurance), in which a single premium payment is converted to a guaranteed monthly income for a specified period of time for the rest of your life. The taxes involved may be complicated and should therefore be vetted with a financial/legal/tax expert to fully understand the implications of the annuity.

## MEDICAID

Medicaid is a state/federal program that assists individuals with low income to pay for health care, including long-term care services and custodial care in a nursing home or at home. One of five individuals in the United States and three of five nursing home residents are covered by Medicaid. The program is administered by each state, so eligibility criteria and services may differ from one state to another after meeting core requirements set by the federal government. In 2017, core requirements included coverage for pregnant women, children, parents, older people, and individuals with disabilities up to specified minimum income levels (based on federal poverty level). States may extend eligibility and have flexibility in promoting their programs, so it is important to learn what the rules and services are in your state. Nursing home care is always covered, but coverage for in-home services varies.

Applications for Medicaid can be obtained from your state office.

---

### QUALIFYING FOR MEDICAID
#### • *The Kiplings' Story* •

Tony was tightly holding Stella's hand and his own jaw. He was not talking, but with muscles tensed and eyes alert, he appeared ready to spring at the slightest provocation. He had just informed the head nurse on the unit that he was leaving and taking Stella with him, never to return. Stella had just moved into the unit two weeks earlier. For the past eight years, Tony had cared for her every need at home, managing with the help of only one other paid caregiver. Tony had watched the facility's staff fumble with understanding Stella's needs as they got to know her. Although the staff had called him numerous times with questions or reports to keep him involved and provide the best care, each call increased his regret that he had moved her into a facility. The final straw came when he received the bill for 45 days of care and understood the status of her Medicaid application would not be known for at least 90 days.

The three of us sat on a couch, with Stella tucked in close next to Tony. Tony was seething and working to regain his composure. Finally, it all came tumbling out. "They don't know her here. They think she is having seizures but she just shakes a little. They want tests, but she's fine. Who's going to pay for all these tests? Is it going to be added to my bill? Everything else is. How am I going to pay for this? I'm such a mess, I can't even work. If I can't work, how am I going to pay for all this? What if Medicaid decides they won't pick up the cost—then will I have to go bankrupt? Will I lose my house? I can't take any more of this. We are better off home together."

---

Meeting eligibility qualifications is the most confusing aspect of understanding Medicaid. Most individuals obtain assistance from an eldercare lawyer or a local social worker. Those who need and access care via Medicaid are as pleased with their care as those who use private insurance. The access to care is good, with a few exceptions (for example, dentists and psychiatrists). Core benefits include physician services, laboratory, and X-ray services, inpatient hospital services, nursing facility services for those 21 or older, home health services for those entitled to nursing facility care, plus a number of other services important for those with conditions other than dementia.

Many individuals (or couples) find that they do not qualify for Medicaid because of their current level of income or assets. The process of "spending down" begins as their assets are used for medical care. Again, discussing these issues with a lawyer or social worker who specializes in eldercare issues specific to the state you live in is strongly recommended. The services of these individuals can help in avoiding delays or inadvertently becoming ineligible because of a financial mistake. There are divestiture rules that are important to discuss with a financial expert and follow closely.

The Kipling family was worried about losing their house, as one spouse needed skilled care and the other did not. The home is exempt if a spouse or disabled child lives there—it is an asset if the applicant does not plan to return there. Other exemptions include furnishings and other personal belongings, one car, prepaid burial assets, and a life insurance policy with a relatively low face value (face values may vary by state). To avoid spousal impoverishment, Medicaid allows the spouse to retain his or her own retirement funds and up to 50 percent of other assets to a maximum that is set every year (to reflect inflation and state differences). The spouse is also entitled to a minimum monthly maintenance allowance from his or her monthly income.

The next issue involves excess monthly income of the individual. Excess monthly income can be used to purchase medical necessities, such as incontinence briefs, if needed. Monthly income may then be eligible for the room and board aspect of long-term care.

*Program of All-Inclusive Care for the Elderly (PACE):* PACE is a Medicare and Medicaid program that provides health care in the community instead of a nursing home for individuals who qualify for nursing home level of care. Only certain regions have PACE programs. PACE coordinates care with a care manager who gets to know a person and his or her family and then works to find the best care and services in the community to meet the individual's needs. The financial model for PACE depends on the individual's resources but has a monthly premium (except for those on Medicaid). Several services not covered by Medicare may be covered in a PACE program. Check with your Medicare office to explore these options.

*Social Security Disability Insurance (SSDI) and Supplemental Security Insurance (SSI)*: SSDI provides benefits to disabled or blind persons who are "insured" by the workers' contributions to the Social Security trust fund. These contributions are based on the workers' earnings (or those of your spouse or parents) as required by the Federal Insurance Contributions Act (FICA). Title II of the Social Security Act authorizes SSDI benefits. Your dependents may also be eligible for benefits from your earnings record.

The SSI program makes payments to those aged 65 or older, blind, or disabled (including children) who have limited income and resources. Even though Social Security manages the program, SSI is not paid for by Social Security taxes. SSI is paid for by US Treasury general funds, not the Social Security trust funds. Many states pay a supplemental benefit to individuals in addition to their federal benefits. Some of these states have made arrangements to combine their supplemental payment with the federal SSI payment, so that you receive one monthly check. Other states manage their own programs and make their payments separately. Title XVI of the Social Security Act authorizes SSI benefits.

The Compassionate Allowances (CAL) initiative is a way to expedite the processing of SSDI and SSI disability claims for applicants whose medical conditions are so severe that their conditions obviously meet Social Security's definition of disability. It is not a separate program from the Social Security Administration's two disability programs, SSDI and SSI.

## ESTATE CLOSING AFTER DEATH

The loss of a family member is a time of emotional upheaval, and a period of clouded thinking is common. I am not uncommonly asked by a spouse caregiver if he or she may now be developing dementia. Usually, this muddled thinking is a grief reaction after a family member passes. Unfortunately, this is a time when a host of legal and financial activities must take place. Trusted individuals are your best resources at this time, as you are likely to need the services of an accountant, an attorney, a clergy, or a grief counselor to assist with the emotional, legal, and financial issues that come with the death of a family member.

I remember accompanying my mother to various banks after my father's death. I came to understand the importance of a joint account so that she could continue to pay bills and attend to day-to-day tasks while issues were being decided in probate court. I also remember my mother cashing a life insurance check issued to her and, in her grief, not clearly handling the matter. Predeath preparation or identifying a trusted individual during this time of intense financial and legal activity is important.

### Probate

Probate is the act or process of proving a will is valid and reflects the wishes of a deceased individual, identifying and inventorying a decedent's property, paying any taxes and debts, and distributing the remainder to the beneficiaries named in the will or according to state law. The probate process is a template that guides the transfer of an estate according to specific rules created by each state.

Probate may vary according to state law but proceeds along the following general lines. A will names or the court appoints an executor, or personal representative, who files papers with the local probate court. Most executors obtain the assistance of an attorney to guide them through the local probate process. The executor assembles all assets that the decedent owned (stocks, bonds, accounts at any and all financial institutions, insurance policies, annuities, property, etc.) and manages these assets during the probate process. For example, the executor may need to obtain an employer identification number for the estate from the IRS, open an estate account, post estate bond, or pay taxes. The executor then identifies any outstanding debts that the decedent may have. Finally, the executor notifies beneficiaries and creditors that the decedent has passed away.

Creditors are then paid out of the estate funds (and properties as assets), after which the beneficiaries receive anything that may have been left to them. Once the court is satisfied that all creditors have been paid, all beneficiaries and assets have been identified, and all taxes have been paid, it grants the executor permission to divide the remaining assets among the people named in the will.

### POINTS TO REMEMBER

▸ The key to making legal and financial decisions rests in values, about life and your hopes, dreams, and fears about the end stage of your disease. The Conversation Project Starter Kit can be helpful in outlining these goals.

▸ A durable power of attorney for health care is a document that lets you name someone else to make decisions about your health care in case you are not able to make those decisions yourself. A lawyer is not required to establish a durable power of attorney but should probably be consulted if you plan to establish one. There are nuances that should be considered about what authorities you will relinquish and when.

▸ A guardian is a person, institute, or agency appointed by a court to manage someone's personal affairs, such as finances, housing, and medical decisions. Guardianship is a serious matter that intrudes on personal liberties and is therefore considered as a last resort when other alternatives have not been successful. Other forms of assistance such as living wills, trusts, case management, and powers of attorney are more common and preferred ways of providing appropriate assistance to someone who is living with dementia.

▶ Advance directives are written instructions that provide information on your goals and wishes if you were seriously ill, dying, or living with a long-term chronic, disabling condition such as Alzheimer disease or related dementias. They are prepared when an individual has mental capacity.

▶ The POLST conversation is about the disease, treatment options and alternatives, and what the patient would want done based on his or her goals of care and values. After the conversation, the health care provider fills out a POLST form, marking what treatments can be chosen (or not chosen) at the end of your life.

▶ The host of programs and insurance options to pay for long-term or end-of-life care include Medicare, Medicaid, private health insurance, long-term care insurance, Social Security Disability Insurance, and Supplemental Security Insurance. Use the websites of each program to guide your search and address your questions.

▶ Estate closing often needs to be dealt with through a probate process. Each state has individual probate processes. Most executors obtain the assistance of an attorney to guide them through the local probate process.

————————————————  ACTION PLAN  ————————————————

▶ Download the tool kit at conversationproject.org. Share with family members and other decision makers to facilitate conversations for goals of care.

▶ Query friends, the Area Agency on Aging, and geriatric specialists for the names of reputable elder law attorneys to assist with legal and financial issues. Check with the local bar association that the attorney is in good standing. Before hiring a lawyer, ask for and check references. Be sure to review and ask for a full explanation of the retainer agreement before committing to working with the lawyer.

## ADDITIONAL READING AND RESOURCES

Few books are available to guide you on the legal and financial aspects of end-of-life care in older adults with dementia. Various government websites seem to offer the best, reliable, and most up-to-date information.

▶ Alzheimers.gov

This website, also sponsored by the Department of Health and Human Services, covers information and educational material on definitions and types of dementia, treatment options, planning strategies for care, finances and housing, community support, and advocacy information. There are several helpful cross-links to other government websites, such as the Veterans Administration, to assist in planning care strategies.

▶ LongTermCare.gov

This website, sponsored by the Department of Health and Human Services, uses graphics, simple statistics, and an easy-to-follow interface to begin the process of understanding long-term care: what it is, who will need it, types of long-term care, costs, and how to pay for it. Several cross-linked websites provide additional resources to understand specifics in more depth for individual families.

▶ Medicare.gov

The Medicare website is relatively easy to navigate and includes information on plans, costs, coverage, appeals, supplemental coverage, and health issues. It also has easy-to-use search features, comparisons, quality metrics, and contact information.

# 5

# Complex Medical Decisions

Dementia is an incurable disease. The final stages are characterized by increasing severe disability, and medical decisions tend to become more and more complex. Making an accurate assessment of prognosis is difficult in advanced dementia, but recent work has described (using a Global Deterioration Scale) that average survival time is a little over a year once profound memory deficits, minimal verbal ability, inability to walk independently, inability to care for daily activities, and incontinence of bowel and bladder have developed. When the decline has reached this level, family and caregivers opt for and value focusing on comfort, rather than on survival.

---

## DECIDING ON A LIMITED APPROACH
### • The Kenny Family Story •

The heavy snow felled trees that took out scores of power lines all over New England; the power outages lasted over a week. The assisted living facility was running on an emergency generator, but still the routines were altered. Meals were simpler, staffing was limited. My mother, who was spending upward of 20 hours per day asleep, sensed the change and decided to close her mouth to any more food. She was shrinking, eating less and less each day. The hospice nurse called to tell me, though I could see it for myself. My mother's forehead folded and furrowed when someone put a spoon to her lips; for me the signs were more subtle, she set her lips into a thin line. We all slowly honored her wishes, briefly offering food but backing off when she showed us her signals for "no thank you." Her trips to the dining room were to watch me interact with her neighbors rather than to eat. At times she would smile at my antics to entertain the room, but mostly she just watched us as if we were behind glass, removed from her. Once she decided to stop eating completely, she passed peacefully within the month.

This was the final limit on medical interventions for my mother. We had foregone treatment for her atrial fibrillation and high blood pressure; the medical interventions designed to prevent strokes were ineffective. We withheld antibiotics for urinary tract infections because they only caused abdominal pain and diarrhea. For the episode of pneumonia that prompted the call to hospice, sleep, sips of water when awake, and cough syrup were used to treat symptoms rather than antibiotics or a hospitalization. Because of our limited medical approach, my mother suffered few of the medically induced side effects I've witnessed in other individuals with dementia. I believe she ultimately benefited from the palliative approach and hospice care that focused exclusively on symptom management.

---

Disability is severe and continues to increase in the final stages of dementia. Health care providers should guide families about the disease trajectory but, unfortunately, often do not. Whether this is due to lack of understanding of the end-of-life course in dementia, their personal discomfort with death, or the focus on cure in their training is unclear. When health care providers do not provide guidance, families find it helpful to learn about the disease and understand their options to make decisions on their own.

---

## RECOGNIZING ADVANCED STAGES
• *The Turning Family Story* •

Joyce, wrapped in a heavy winter coat, a hat, and a blanket, was surrounded by her family. The heavy covering did not conceal the bones of her cheeks, a vacant stare, and a slackened jaw. She was having trouble keeping her eyes open. Joyce's two sons, a daughter, and a daughter-in-law all looked worried. One son was angry and impatient as he picked at his eyebrow and looked quickly back and forth between his mother and me.

The Turnings were concerned their mother might have another urinary tract infection as she was sleepier than usual. Although Joyce had a primary care physician and was scheduled to see a geriatrician the next week, the family had pleaded for an "emergency appointment" because of her change in status. Joyce's daughter began, telling me that her mother had been diagnosed with dementia eight years ago, had been home with help the entire time, and had 24-hour care between paid aides and family for the last two years. Joyce was losing weight no matter how carefully she was being fed, and repeated infections caused her to lapse into near comatose states, requiring hospitalization that always resulted in delirium and extreme agitation. One of the sons, Tom, had been squirming while his sister told the story and finally growled loudly, "What are we supposed to do? This is crazy!"

I asked whether they had discussed advance directives and long-term care plans before. Joyce's daughter said, "Yes, we don't want her resuscitated if her heart stops. We have that document." Tom kept muttering while Joyce's other son and daughter-in-law inched away from him. "OK, how about long-term plans?" I asked. Tom blew, raising his voice and speaking in punctuated sentences. "What choice do we have? What can we do? This is terrible. We treat each setback only to make her worse. We're losing her." Tom's jaw clenched, and he started to cry. I responded, "I can see that you've provided the best care possible for your mom. She has all your love and support. She has been home and is comfortable. But she is reaching a point that you *are* losing her. I'm sorry if I'm the first one to tell you this." The other siblings also began to tear up, but we were able to have an open and honest discussion about the next steps and goals of care for Joyce in her final phase of living and dying with dementia.

---

## PERSON-CENTERED APPROACH TO CARE

We have discussed the principles of making decisions for others (chapter 3) for care in the advanced stage of dementia. The level and type of care should be guided by goals agreed on by the surrogate decision maker and the care providers as a team. Care providers can outline the typical course with treatment options so that families can make the best decisions for the individual. Few treatment options have been evaluated in studies of individuals with advanced dementia, so recommendations and decisions must be made from what we do know or can extrapolate from available information.

Individual autonomy and well-being are often balanced (or not balanced) with safety as others take on the responsibility for individuals who have lost the capacity to decide for themselves. Remaining focused on the perceived or stated wishes of the person in our approach to care (that is, taking what is called a person-centered approach) is helpful, but the level of comfort with risk management varies among surrogate decision makers. Can an individual put personal risk aversion aside when deciding on the course of action that would make his or her family member most comfortable? A dear patient of mine loved going for walks in the woods behind her house. During this solitary time in the surroundings of nature, she felt grounded and reflected on her feelings and thoughts. But as her gait became unsteady, her husband began to forbid her forest walks, and she fell into a depression. Recognizing this, her husband started accompanying her on the walks, but part of her need and joy in the woods had been her solitude and quiet reflective time. Her husband adapted by walking her to a bench they'd placed in the forest and finding the courage to leave her sitting there alone. He was terrified she would stand up, walk, and fall or become lost. He found if he didn't leave her though, she suffered in other ways. Putting her well-being first, he decided to enter therapy to learn to deal with the panic this risk caused him. When I jokingly suggested he outfit her in a bright neon orange cap so that he could spot her from afar, he did just that! He reported it was a godsend as he could see the orange cap, safe, and sound at the bench site, while she was able to enjoy her time of quiet and solitude.

## COMMON CONDITIONS WITH ALTERNATIVE APPROACHES TO CARE

### Eating, Feeding, and Nutrition

The most common complication of advancing dementia is in eating, occurring in approximately 90 percent of those living with late-stage dementia. In addition to not being able to coordinate the act of bringing food to one's mouth, issues such as "pocketing" food in the cheeks, coughing and choking with swallowing, and refusing to eat are common scenarios.

### Weight Loss or Just Less Food Intake?

In evaluating changes in eating, first we must decide whether there is a problem. Is there weight loss? The loss of appetite may be due to decreased energy output. If there is little movement or physical activity, not as much food is required. What seems like not enough to live on may be an adequate amount for that individual. If there is no weight loss, simply monitoring for safe, nutritious food choices without concern over the small amount of food consumed may be enough.

My mom went through a phase of eating less and some weight loss after an acute illness during her middle stages of dementia. She, along with our family for support, used several strategies to increase her caloric and nutritional intake so that she could regain some weight. But in her late stages, when she had nearly stopped walking, her need for food was less. While it was a bit hard not to nudge her to have another bite or two at meals, she was listening to her body and really didn't need any more food. When I forgot and pushed a little more so that she complied, she would either feel sick the rest of the night or get angry at me without really understanding why. I only understood in retrospect that her anger was a signal that I shouldn't have been quite so insistent on pushing the food.

## PROBLEMS WITH CHEWING AND SWALLOWING FOOD

Has eating become difficult? Think about the entire eating process. Can your family member still manage using utensils? Would it be helpful to obtain specialized utensils that can be more easily used by someone who has arthritis or memory loss? Do dentures fit? Are there sores in the mouth or teeth that need a dentist's attention? Is there any difficulty with swallowing or choking? Many conditions accompany aging and dementia that may make eating difficult. A checkup with the physician or dentist with your observations and direct questions is in order. My mother had a short period where nothing tasted good to her. She couldn't quite tell us why nothing tasted good, but she shied away from many foods. Eventually, I realized that she wasn't able to properly perform mouth care. Food was getting stuck around the teeth in the back of her mouth, and the yeast infection that developed had affected her taste for food. Once we treated the infection and began assisting with mouth care, her appetite bounced right back.

If eating issues persist once any reversible causes have been attended to, choices on how to approach the change in eating can be addressed. There is little research evidence to warrant the use of medications or diet modification to improve function or survival, so choosing a treatment to attempt to prolong life is not helpful.

### Issues with Feeding Tubes

So, what *can* help? I am often asked about tube feeding. Reviews of tube feeding in people with advanced dementia have not found it to be beneficial, as defined by survival, nutrition, prevention of aspiration pneumonia, or healing of pressure ulcers. In fact, tube feeding may even be harmful because of associated risks. A surgical procedure is required to insert the tube, and bleeding or infection can result. After the tube is in place, individuals commonly go back and forth to the emergency room for tube difficulties, such as the tube becoming clogged or pulled out accidentally. Several health care groups have made public recommendations *against* tube feeding based on evidence and expert opinion, including the American Board of Internal Medicine, American Geriatrics Society, American Academy of Hospice and Palliative Medicine, and the Alzheimer's Association.

---

### UNDERSTANDING PROGNOSIS
#### • *The William Family Story* •

Melinda and Scott were sipping coffee from disposable cups when I walked in. They both had eyes half closed and looked exhausted. We had been planning to meet next week to discuss Oscar's prognosis and plan of care, but they had flown into town earlier than expected to deal with Melinda's mother, who had been physically declining and was now acutely hospitalized. Melinda had just taken on the decision making for her father and asked for a palliative care consult. Oscar had been eating less and losing weight. He was coughing after any food intake. He hadn't walked independently in over a year, and he'd had three fainting spells when on the toilet. Oscar was on a host of medicines. Melinda wanted to discuss Oscar's prognosis, medications, and plan of care. She pulled out a list of questions: "Why is my dad on cholesterol medicines? Will they help him? And he is on two blood pressure medicines, but he has been fainting. Could they be too much? I'm told he is losing weight—is this normal or should something be done? I know he doesn't want a feeding tube, but are there other options and do they work? How often should he go to the hospital to get food or fluids if he keeps getting dehydrated or losing weight?"

I commended Melinda on her thoughtful list. We backed the discussion up to the prognosis, and I confirmed that Oscar was in the end stage of dementia and would qualify for hospice as a potential option. Knowing that Oscar's dementia was advanced helped answer questions about medications. Because cholesterol-lowering agents and blood pressure medication are used to help prevent heart attack and stroke, they likely would not be beneficial to Oscar and may indeed be contributing to his loss of appetite and fainting spells. We talked of his weight loss. Yes, this is normal with advancing dementia. We discussed how dehydration is also normal with end-stage diseases, including dementia, and that this allows the body to comfortably shut down without excess secretions, sweating, urination, and defecation. Melinda looked at me quizzically. "Don't we have to feed him? Are we starving him?" We discussed that food is an emotionally charged topic. Food has so many meanings. It is the fuel our body needs to function, but we have a more personal, often spiritual, connection to food. In times of both sickness and celebration, we gather around food. But when a disease has progressed to end stages, loss of appetite and weight loss are a normal part of preparing for death, and it is perfectly fine to allow this to occur without medical intervention. Melinda and I discussed ways she could be with her father and focus on the personal, spiritual connection itself rather than on food.

Melinda sat back and said, "It seems there is no need to have my father hospitalized now. He can stay here, surrounded by people who know and love him and will take good care of him." I wholeheartedly agreed.

---

## THE LAST STAGE AND RISK OF ASPIRATION

Most health care providers specializing in approaches to care for those with dementia recommend hand feeding. The goals of hand feeding are many, including to provide food for pleasure and comfort and to provide contact and interaction with another person. The feeding may still result in aspiration, but when someone is aspirating small amounts of carefully offered food, they likely are also aspirating secretions from their mouth. Unfortunately, this cannot be avoided as part of the late stages of dementia, when the throat muscles can no longer successfully protect *anything* that leaves the mouth from entering the airway. Offering food is for the taste and pleasure, done to provide a quality of life, not to provide fuel to prolong life.

## Antibiotics and Infections

### FOCUSING ON COMFORT, RATHER THAN ON TREATMENT, WHEN DYING WITH DEMENTIA
#### • *The Russo Family Story* •

Anger and frustration were building between Abigail, her daughter, Barbara, and the nursing staff. On several occasions, Barbara reported her mother's chattiness and thick speech to the nurses as evidence of an impending infection, but the nurses needed more objective signs and symptoms before calling a physician for an evaluation and possibly new orders. When the infection would "hit," Barbara was angry and frustrated that it hadn't been dealt with days or weeks before. Likewise, the nurses felt frustrated because they were being blamed for neglect when there was no objective medical evidence of infection such as fever, rapid heart rate, rapid breathing, or sleepiness. On my review of the situation, I saw Abigail as progressively failing over the last year due to her dementia. She was sleeping more hours of the day, she was having repeat infections, she had lost the ability to walk independently, and she was participating less and less in her surroundings. When I spoke with Abigail, she awoke, made beautiful, deep eye contact, and smiled. I told her I was going to meet with her daughter. She said "Karen" and I said, "No, Barbara is coming." She smiled and nodded back off to sleep. I felt Abigail's warm, gentle energy and understood why Barbara fought so hard to maintain her mother's health. But dementia was taking her life. I sat with Barbara and Payton, Abigail's son, and asked them to describe their understanding of Abigail's condition. Barbara began telling me of her mother's course over the last few years, her ability to intuit changes in her mother's condition and her frustration that she wasn't heard or her opinion honored.

Payton spoke up and said, "Honestly, I see my mother failing. She can be bright with me for a few minutes, but when I walk in and watch her from afar, it is so sad how she has gotten so small and seems gone. I know I'm not here as much as Barbara, but I don't think this is what my mom would have wanted." Barbara was tearing up at hearing Payton's words. "I've wondered how we would know if Mom is going. I know I'm tired, but does that mean it's time to give up?" I acknowledged that there were signs that Abigail had turned a corner and was now dying with dementia, rather than living with dementia. Payton reached out and took Barbara's hand. Both were now openly crying. Payton continued, "Let's change our plans and help Mom and our kids with this. I like that as a way to explain . . . she is dying with dementia now. We helped her live with it. This will help us make decisions and be able to tell the kids." Barbara looked tenderly at Payton and heard him. She started to see the situation in a new light. This opened the conversation to how to address the infections. Barbara talked about how, without antibiotics, we might support her mother when she noticed chattiness, thick speech, or any other symptom. We discussed how she could advocate for her mother and work with the nurses on controlling symptoms—and that much of this would not require medical intervention but human interventions. Barbara's advocacy now had an ear; Abigail's family would assist her in comfortably dying.

---

Infections, usually of the urinary tract or the lungs (pneumonia), occur in approximately two-thirds of individuals during their last year of life. Death from any cause occurs within six months in more than half of individuals with late-stage dementia who are diagnosed with pneumonia. These statistics show us that infection is part of a larger picture of the frailty and decline that accompany the late stage of dementia. Why do those with dementia have infections? A host of reasons: the immune system is impaired due to age and diminished nutrition, the dementia disease process impairs ability to cough to clear the airway or avoid mouth secretions from entering the lungs, urine flow is decreased impairing the ability to clear bacteria from the urinary tract. What then is a reasonable approach to infections? It depends on the goals of care. Is the goal to prolong life, focus on comfort, or strike a balance between the two? Understanding the pros and cons of each approach can help in making this decision.

Focusing on comfort means treating symptoms, regardless of presence of infection. For example, if there is a fever, treatment would be to bring the fever down by using medications, placing a cool compress on the forehead, or providing a cool drink to sip. If shortness of breath develops, oxygen, a fan over the face, and/or medication such as morphine to help with the sense of breathlessness may be provided. Any type of infection can cause pain. For pain management, the first step is to be aware of typical signs of pain, which include restlessness, agitation, grimacing, moaning, and calling out, and then to address with the appropriate level of pain control.

The benefit, therefore, of symptom relief is that symptoms are well controlled and diagnostic testing is avoided. The risk of symptom relief is that the infections may result in further sickness that may shorten life. In a study on survival and comfort in individuals with advanced dementia who had pneumonia, those who received antibiotics lived approximately nine months longer than those who did not, but there was more reported discomfort. In contrast, there is no evidence that providing antibiotics for a urinary tract infection prolongs survival in those with advanced dementia. What is known is that *suspected* urinary tract infections often receive antibiotics (81% of the time) when there is no clear evidence of a meaningful infection, so that overtreatment with antibiotics of noninfections is the norm.

## Benefits and Risks of Antibiotics

What are the benefits of providing antibiotics? Antibiotics treat infections caused by bacteria; antiviral medications treat infections caused by viruses. The benefits of antibiotics are treatment of infection, thereby curing it or keeping it from spreading. However, the use of antibiotics also has risks; they may be used when they are not warranted and may result in serious side effects. A rash (that may be as extensive as a severe burn), diarrhea, nausea, and fever are the most common.

To avoid administering antibiotics when they are not warranted, testing for the infection is required. This may mean testing the blood or urine. When antibiotics are given without adequate testing, suspected infections are overtreated; this is the common scenario in those with advanced dementia because testing can be burdensome. This overtreatment is playing into antibiotic-resistant bacteria surviving and thriving, causing what is termed *superinfections*. We are now facing a skilled nursing facility, if not national, crisis of multi-drug-resistant organisms, which makes treatment of verified infections more and more difficult. The percentage of individuals with advanced dementia living in a skilled facility with antibiotic-resistant colonization of their nose, bladder, or other mucosa is approximately 66 percent. Frequent hospitalization spreads the resistant strains of organisms to others in the hospital and community.

## Testing for Infections

To adequately test urine for an infection, sterile techniques need to be followed, such as cleaning the genital area just before voiding and then catching the urine in the middle of the stream. If this cannot be done, for example, when someone cannot follow these directions or void when asked, as is common in those with dementia, catheterization is required to obtain an adequate sample. However, catheterization is not without risk. It can *cause* infection if performed without sterile technique or if insertion of the catheter causes minor injury to the fragile tissue of the urethra. For these reasons, suspicion of infection is often cause for antibiotics to be initiated, though warranted less than 20 percent of the time by clinical criteria. Further, older adults often have urinary tracts colonized with bacteria (meaning the bacteria are living in the tract but not causing an infectious process), making the decision to treat even more difficult when faced with a positive culture and vague symptoms. Colonization is especially likely to occur in those with advanced dementia—three times more likely than in those without dementia. Clinical criteria may be used to assist in the decision to treat or not, but the criteria for urinary tract infections depend heavily on reported symptoms, which are unreliable in the typically nonverbal individual with advanced dementia.

Testing for pneumonia (via symptoms such as fever, cough, and rapid breathing rate and positive radiologic findings) is more accurate than testing for urinary tract infection. Even so, the proportion of respiratory infections meeting minimum clinical criteria is only about a third, and overtreatment is still the rule.

Side effects from antibiotic use in frail, older individuals with late-stage dementia cannot be clearly identified and may be difficult to test for. It may also be difficult to determine whether symptoms that are recognized are due to antibiotics. Diarrhea following antibiotic use is reported to occur in approximately 45 percent of those in nursing homes. Side effects such as nausea and loss of appetite are difficult to quantify in those with limited ability to communicate. When my older, frail, but cognitively intact patients reported these problems, it helped me understand some of these more subtle, albeit real, side effects. Several individuals told me they couldn't finish a course of antibiotics because of nausea, loss of appetite, abdominal cramping, insomnia, and achiness. Despite the fact that this "evidence" is only anecdotal, my many years of practice focusing on adults older than 80 instilled a respect for the potential harmful side effects of antibiotic treatment.

The use of antibiotics for vague symptoms in older adults living with dementia is the norm. Whether this is driven by health care providers or caregivers is not clear. What is known is that only 33 percent of family members are counseled by health care prescribers on the common outcome of infection in dementia. When these conversations do occur, overtreatment of vague symptoms with antibiotics is less common.

# PREVENTIVE AND DISEASE-MODIFYING TREATMENTS FOR OTHER CHRONIC DISEASES

## USING WELL-BEING AS A GUIDE TO TESTING AND INTERVENTIONS IN LATE-STAGE DEMENTIA

• *The Jensen Family Story* •

Mr. Jensen moved to a facility after two months of bouncing back and forth between the hospital and rehabilitation sites. His frail wife and three devoted children, Laurie, Anna, and Oliver, had been sitting with him, often day and night, during these past months. They tried to assist, comfort, and calm him, as each transition wreaked havoc on his mental state. Laurie described her father's cognitive condition over the last year, knowing that we were currently dealing with delirium while I hoped to gauge his prior stage of dementia.

In the 10 months leading up to his repeated hospitalizations, he had been losing the ability to speak, sleeping more, and interacting less. He had begun to lose weight, not because of swallowing difficulty, but because he slept through most meals and wasn't interested in food when it was offered. Her father had two known cancers, both in quiet states, but enlarged lymph nodes recently found in his abdomen were suggestive of a new cancer. The family had chosen not to further evaluate the nodes because "my dad is so old, his thinking is already off and these hospitalizations are so hard on him." We talked further so I could understand how the family felt about medical interventions, in light of the advancing dementia and possible third cancer. Laurie wanted to learn more about dementia. We discussed that dementia is a terminal disease but, much like cancer, can have a long period of chronicity in which life is lived well, with some adaptation but reasonable function. Also similar to cancer, when dementia progresses further with more prevalent signs and symptoms, letting go of medical interventions may be the best way to live life well and allow for a natural death.

Laurie, using her father's cancers to guide her thinking, acknowledged that her father's dementia had advanced, but she wasn't sure to what degree. Although we would work on addressing the delirium, the family could still decide to limit their father's care once his stage of dementia was better defined. "We've all been grappling with doing too much or too little. It is comforting to know that we may not know. It is also comforting to know one decision can be made now and others can be considered later. I've been so caught up in having answers, I failed to see that not knowing was OK."

---

The continued treatment of chronic disease states and prevention of disease is an often asked question when dementia is approached from a palliative lens. Many family members and sometimes even physicians ask why I bother "upsetting the apple cart." The number and type of medications often used with advancing age and near end of life can be quite burdensome. With dementia, this burden increases even more. Every medication carries the risk of drug-drug interactions, and any medication or intervention has potential adverse reactions. Just administering—and taking—medications can be troublesome. I sat at my mother's table in the dining room, watching the other residents struggle with the bitter taste of crushed medications before eating. No wonder many lost their appetite by the time food was offered.

## Medications to Prevent Disease

A systematic approach can be helpful to many families as they wrestle with these questions. For treatments that prevent disease, discontinuing treatment is relatively easy. Because medications used to prevent a heart attack or stroke decrease risk over the long term, there is no acute harm to stopping them. Few studies have addressed this directly, but one that looked at statin medications, which are used to lower cholesterol, found that discontinuation was safe and resulted in improved well-being. This suggests that treatments for high cholesterol, blood pressure, and stroke prevention may be discontinued in the vast majority of individuals.

## Medications That Treat an Established Chronic Condition

What about when the medication is being used to treat a condition? The condition that comes to mind is dementia itself. Is there a place for medications used to treat dementia when the disease is in its final stage? A consensus of 12 geriatric and palliative care specialists felt there was no continued benefit to using these medications in late stages of dementia. Similarly, treating high blood pressure is likely no longer necessary, because the goals of treating are to deter long-term problems with the kidneys, heart, or brain.

I was recently asked about whether to continue cystoscopy in a gentleman with a history of bladder cancer to monitor for recurrence. His life expectancy was less than a year due to his late-stage dementia. His family would not have reinstituted treatment for bladder cancer if it recurred, so the value of the procedure was questionable at best. He had no symptoms of bladder trouble—no blood, no evidence of pain, no difficulty with urine flow. I recommended surveillance via cystoscopy be discontinued, and the family readily agreed.

## Questions to Help in Decisions about Medications

To assist in making decisions about the treatments or procedures to be continued near the end of life, I find that asking a series of questions helps. Will stopping the treatment cause immediate harm? Can it provide relief? Will undergoing testing change the course of care? If not, is there any other reason to perform the test? Questions like these can help family members sort out many situations. For example, what should be done if an individual has a hip fracture? Transfer to the hospital for surgical intervention may be warranted to limit pain in someone who is relatively active, but for someone who remains in bed, treatment with pain medications may be the better alternative.

## TRANSFER TO HOSPITAL

When medical conditions escalate, a transfer to the hospital is the typical response. But does it have to be? The most common causes for hospital transfer of individuals with late-stage dementia are infections, although other acute flare-ups of chronic conditions (such as lung disease or heart failure) can also warrant admission. If a feeding tube is part of the care plan, nearly half of emergency room transfers are to deal with unanticipated complications, such as dislodging or blockages.

### Risk and Benefits of Hospitalization

The benefits of hospitalization in late-stage dementia are unclear. Hospitalizations are rife with burdensome and costly testing and interventions, accounting for 30 percent of Medicare expenditures. Hospital settings, overall, are not without major risk to those with advanced dementia; delirium nearly always develops, resulting in either physical or medical restraints that may then result in bed sores, aspirations, psychological stress, and potentially death. Caregiver burden, psychological stress, and increased depression have been reported with the decision for nursing home admission. I have also witnessed that the trauma of an acute hospitalization causes further distress to the family caregiver who watches the delirium and often receives medical advice, at times conflicting, from multiple health care professionals.

### Advance Care Planning to Address Potential Conditions Commonly Causing Hospitalization

Advance care planning can help minimize hospitalizations. Respiratory infections are the most common cause for transfer to hospitals, but this condition can be managed as well in a skilled nursing facility or home. If goals of care (prolongation of life versus comfort) are discussed before an acute illness, a more comfortable approach may be taken. My mother was able to remain in her assisted living facility, without a single hospitalization, in her last two years of life, despite urinary tract infections, pneumonias, weight loss, and other common illnesses as her dementia progressed. I believe she avoided many side effects of medications or medical procedures.

## PALLIATIVE AND HOSPICE CARE

*Hospice* is a term used both for a palliative approach to care and a health care benefit. A palliative approach is care that focuses on the comfort and dignity of the individual in his or her final months of life and includes families and caregivers. The focus is usually on alleviating pain or other distressing symptoms, while supporting living, rather than on treating or trying to cure the underlying condition. Because pain or discomfort can be physical, mental, spiritual, or existential, the hospice approach requires a team that includes those with expertise in medicine (physician, nurses, and health aides), counseling (social workers, counselors, and clergy), and respite (volunteers, family). A recent review of 43 randomized controlled trials of palliative care found that a palliative approach improved quality of life, decreased the burden of disease symptoms, and improved advance care planning and patient and caregiver satisfaction.

---
### POINTS TO REMEMBER

▶ Dementia is an incurable disease; a shift in focus of care to comfort in the final stage is appropriate.

▶ An alternative to a curative or supportive approach to care is a palliative or symptom-focused approach.

▶ Nutrition or eating can shift to offering food for pleasure rather than for life-sustaining nutritional needs. The focus can remain on gathering around food for community and love, rather than on the nutritional needs of the body.

▶ In those with end-stage dementia, treatment of infections with antibiotics does not prolong life significantly, if at all. Treatment of symptoms, such as fever, shortness of breath, or pain, is a gentle alternative and avoids the potential side effects of antibiotic therapy. Discontinuing medications for treatment of chronic diseases or to prevent disease is fitting at the end of life with dementia. The burden of medication use is avoided, and medications used to treat symptoms can be prioritized.

▶ Hospitalizations at the end of life are common but result in excess burden, interventions, trauma, complications, and cost. Most palliative care can be delivered from home or other place of residence with comfort and improved quality of life.

───────────────── **ACTION PLAN** ─────────────────

▶ If your family member has entered the last phase of dementia, begin or continue discussions with all involved in decision making to establish goals of care—life sustaining or palliative—and set a time frame appropriate to revisit (monthly, semiannually, after each hospitalization) the goals of care with family members.

▶ Review areas in which an approach may be modified—eating, infections, medications for chronic diseases, hospitalizations, and use of palliative care. Ask yourself: Will stopping the treatment/approach cause immediate harm? Can the treatment/approach provide relief? Will undergoing testing or continuing the approach change the course of care? If not, is there any other reason to perform the test or to continue the approach?

───────────── **ADDITIONAL READINGS AND RESOURCES** ─────────────

▶ *Dementia beyond Disease*, by G. Allen Power, MD

Dr. Power proposes a focus on well-being for those living with dementia and the society that supports them. He argues that shifting the lens from a biomedical model to one of an experiential approach will expand and enhance the decisions and care for those living and dying with dementia. He advocates that the true experts of understanding the disease and care needs are those living with dementia and that the rest of us should remain their students. The chapters review domains of well-being: identity, connectedness, security, autonomy, meaning, growth, and joy. The focus on well-being can be addressed to the end of life, allowing for full and contented existence. The chapter on connectedness is especially meaningful as it explores removing the focus from a medical perspective at end of life.

▶ *Ten Thousand Joys and Ten Thousand Sorrows*, by Olivia Ames Hoblitzelle

In this beautiful book of the journey of Alzheimer disease, Hob and his wife, Olivia, are practicing Buddhists when Hob is diagnosed with Alzheimer disease. They make a pact to live each day together as mindfully and honestly as possible, chronicling the joys and sorrows they experienced, together and separately. The book holds a place for acceptance of death and honoring it in a mindful, loving way.

# Decisions about Places of Care

Choosing where to live and how to modify the living situation with the changes that dementia brings is best done early. But this is neither always possible nor always done. Approximately 70 percent of those older than 65 will need some type of long-term care, whether provided in their home by family or paid caregivers or in a program or facility. The number reaches near 100 percent for those who are diagnosed with dementia. This chapter will highlight the living choices and the common issues, compromises, promises, and pitfalls that accompany the different choices of residence options for those living with dementia.

---

### DETERMINING THE RIGHT LIVING ENVIRONMENT
#### • *The Kenny Family Story* •

I boarded the airplane to accompany my mother from the midwestern hospital to live in New England, either with or near me. When I received the call she was in the hospital, I began a search, fast and furious, for the next right place for her to live. I spent nights sitting at the kitchen table with my husband discussing options for converting the dining room into a bedroom and adding a walk-in shower to the first-floor half-bath. How would that affect the family? How would that affect my ability to work? Could I successfully, confidently, and reliably find supplemental home care? Would my mother, the social being that she is, be too isolated in a home setting? Was there an assisted living facility that could accommodate her needs? Did she need a skilled nursing facility? There are at least a hundred different approaches. I had said this to dozens and dozens of other families I had counseled in the past. Now I was facing the decisions for the best route to go. Each path was pregnant with a host of issues, compromises, promises, and pitfalls. For the earlier stages of disease, we had already made the move to assisted living with escalating supplemental support. But my mother's care needs were continuing to climb, and we needed a new approach.

---

Determining what type of long-term care is needed for someone with dementia depends on a host of resources: family and friends, finances, physical and mental condition at time of diagnosis, history of military service, insurance, and the ability of the family to modify the home. And these are only a few of the factors to be considered in determining the best place of residence. Balance is needed to accommodate both the individual and other family members, and that balance should be reevaluated as the disease progresses. Even initially well-thought-out plans may require changes when things are not working out. Sometimes, a new decision is needed for a new place of care, temporary respite, or integrating additional support from outside.

## PLACE OF RESIDENCE

### Home

---

#### MAKING ADAPTATIONS TO SUPPORT LIVING AT HOME
• *John and Jay's Story* •

John, a retired lawyer, had been seeing me for care for approximately 20 years. He had always been a systematic and methodical individual, but now he reported that his memory was slipping. "I'm sure you won't be able to tell, but I certainly can." He was right. Screens and in-depth neuropsychological testing did not catch any deficits, but memory and some executive functioning tests scored only in the average range. John took good care of himself physically. He ate a heart-healthy diet, walked daily, and engaged in strength training and balance exercises. John knew he needed to make plans to live his life the way he wished. He began adapting his home for a gradual transition to living on one floor by expanding the first floor bathroom and modifying the dining room so that, if needed, one day it could serve as a bedroom.

John put enormous thought into whom he might approach to become his caregiver as he declined. He wanted to be sure it was someone he could trust to follow his plan of care and who would respect his wishes and dignity until the end of his life. He invited his middle son, Jay, to live with him. Jay was between jobs and recognized that he had made some poor choices in his life. Jay realized this would allow him an opportunity to repair his relationship with his father, while also being able to spend time and resources on taking online courses toward an advanced degree. John and Jay developed many common interests, sharing care for their dog, exercising together, and planning elaborate meals. As John became less able to participate in these activities and make decisions, the previous common experiences guided Jay in knowing what to do. For example, when John started wandering at night, Jay adjusted the exercise schedule, adopted eyeshades for John, placed a commode next to John's bed, and modified their schedule to eliminate screen time at night. Jay worked on communication and nonpharmacologic approaches to each troublesome behavior that arose and deftly made changes, with excellent results.

Jay found respite in other family members and in his schooling. John was able to avoid medications as he continued to decline. John moved into the dining room as his ability to walk vanished. Jay was an understanding care partner and approached John's feeding and personal care with patience and love. The family continued weekly gatherings to support John and provide social support to Jay. John died peacefully at home six years after Jay moved in with him.

The desire to live at home is the most common request by individuals with dementia or their families. The benefits to remaining home can be many, but as with any choice, it may also be wrought with troubles. Most people begin their journey with dementia at home but must be willing, along with family, to divert this plan if it is not working out.

## Questions That Aid in Deciding Whether Home Is the Right Fit

It seems it can go without saying that comfort and memories are positive aspects of remaining at home. However, as a physician, I often confront challenges that make staying at home difficult. A good way to approach such decisions is with a series of questions. Does the home accommodate the needs of the individual with cognitive and functional decline? Can getting into and out of the house be done safely? Are there stairs or wheelchair access? Can the individual with limited mobility have access to the outside through windows, porches, or patios? Is the bed accessible, or is it on another floor where an individual with increasing weakness cannot get to?

Are the day-to-day activities of personal care easy to accomplish in the home? Showering or bathing? Dressing? Is there room or ability for those partnering in care to use the bed or the bathroom to assist in care? Can the home be modified to address any of these issues?

Is the person with dementia an introvert or an extrovert? Will the solitude of home be comforting or isolating? Will it be so for the primary caregiver?

I am often surprised at how strongly people fight to remain in their home, even though it may not be in their best interest or the best interest of their caregiver(s). These discussions often happen in earlier stages of dementia, but many individuals have remained home until the late stages of their disease or death.

## Resources Needed to Remain Home

Staying home often depends on resources, adeptness at handling any behaviors that may arise from dementia, and the needs of others living in the home. To combat the isolation that is a common complaint of those at home, contacting volunteer organizations that can provide companionship may be helpful. To assist with the myriad tasks, both to maintain the house and to care for the personal needs of the individual with dementia, help with housework or personal care can be hired or bartered. Most of these services need to be covered with out-of-pocket resources, although there are some grants that may help cover costs (Alzheimer's Foundation of America and the Alzheimer's Association—local, nonprofit member organizations [contact your local office]). When health care needs arise, home care nursing services can be called in to assist with wound care, as an example.

Providing care at home has the benefit of a more holistic care for the individual with dementia, avoiding medical treatments that may not be necessary. But what are the problems and pitfalls of providing care at home? Personal care needs increase with functional loss. Those who assist in the care of a family member with dementia may suffer a financial strain due to lost wages. An emotional strain also may accompany primary caregiving. Finally, there may be isolation, both for the individual with dementia and the primary caregiver. If the strains of caregiving become severe, the caregiver may be at high risk of depression, anxiety, low social contacts, and perceived burden. The risk of abuse and violence also increases.

## Assisted Living or Board and Care Homes

If the care at home is not possible because of troublesome behaviors or because the home cannot be modified to accommodate ongoing needs, assisted living is often an option. Assisted living homes are group living settings that offer housing in addition to assistance with personal care and other services such as transportation, meals, and housekeeping. They usually have 24-hour staff, but some do not.

They are not regulated by the federal government and, therefore, assisted living homes vary from state to state. They usually do not provide medical care, although they may assist with medication and meal reminders or assistance. Some assisted living facilities have special expertise in dementia and provide programming, staff training, and resident support for needs due to dementia. Some assisted living facilities will accommodate aging in place by allowing for individuals and their families to bring in extra, fee-for-service care as dementia progresses and care needs increase.

The services available in assisted living facilities are varied. Similarly, the price structure varies by assisted living site. You should ask questions so that you know what is covered by the daily charge and what other services are available for an extra charge. My mother, for example, first moved to an assisted living facility that required independence in bathing, dressing, toileting, and ambulation. As a family, we knew she would not remain in this setting throughout her journey with dementia. However, she desired this initial move to be near a friend, to have access to a daily religious service on site, and to continue to be able to go places via the robust transportation support provided. Her medications were kept in a clinic and provided to her daily, for an additional fee. My mother hated someone else handling her medications but acquiesced to our concerns when we gently showed her evidence of her inability to successfully manage her medications on her own. This assisted living facility also offered excellent programming for my mother's early level of cognitive decline—there were art and exercises classes, community service projects, book discussion groups, bridge groups, and other excellent opportunities for socialization. As my mother's cognitive abilities declined, she was no longer able to join in these activities, but she was still able to participate in an on-site adult day program. Around this time, unfortunately, my mother began to wander and fall, and we knew her time living in this facility was coming to an end.

We began to explore other assisted living facilities that could accommodate the special needs of those with dementia, such as wandering. We looked for an assisted living environment that would allow her to age in place, by bringing in supplemental care and hospice services when her function declined beyond the resources provided by that assisted living community. Not all facilities accommodate this, which means that another living transition may be needed when care needs increase. The facility we chose had a limitation for lifting—if my mother needed the assistance of more than one person in lifting her for transfers, we would have to provide 24-hour supplemental care. So be sure to check the restrictions of any facilities you are considering before making a move so that you are not surprised later.

### Services and Prices of Assisted Living Facilities Vary: Check Your Family Needs Carefully

AARP (formerly the American Association of Retired Persons) has developed a checklist for evaluating and comparing assisted living facilities (http://assets.aarp.org/www.aarp.org_/promotions/text /life/AssistedLivingChecklist.pdf). Facilities must be vetted for their expertise in dementia care and ability to adapt and accommodate behaviors and functional decline common with dementia. When searching for care that adds special services for those with dementia, questions may be expanded to ask what levels of dementia are supported, who assesses the level of health and cognitive functioning if there are restrictions, what type of support is provided for activities of daily living, what activities are available that are geared to those with memory impairment, and what is the level of training of staff.

Finally, an important consideration in choosing an assisted living facility is the cost. Care in these facilities is rarely covered by insurance. Long-term care insurance may cover some of the amount, but restrictions and deductibles must be met.

## Nursing Facility

---

### CONSIDERING PHYSICAL AND EMOTIONAL
### NEEDS OF THE ENTIRE FAMILY
#### • *The Nowak Family Story* •

Mrs. Nowak and her daughter, Julia, sat bundled in their coats, huddled together, with frightened looks on their faces. We settled into chairs and removed our coats, but the anxious body language remained. Julia began, "My father is failing more and more. Both my parents and my family sold our houses so that we could move into a house with an in-law apartment and be able to help my father as his dementia progressed. But it's too much for all of us. It is too much for me and . . . Mom, please let me say this . . . it's too much for you."

Immediately, Mrs. Nowak began to cry. Julia continued, "My mom is so unhappy having lost her support system in her old town. My father's care needs just keep increasing, and she is wearing herself out. I'm a nurse and I know the facts—she is making herself sick caring for my dad. She needs to . . . we need to consider moving him out of the home, before it kills my mother." I shifted my focus to Mrs. Nowak, handed her a tissue and asked, "What do you think of all this?" "I hear what Julie is saying, but how can I? It feels like . . . " She struggled for the right words. "Abandon?" I asked. Mrs. Nowak looked into my eyes and said, softly and sadly, "Yes. We've been married so long just to leave him at this point. I can do it. I know I can, and then he would feel safe. I just can't imagine how he'd feel when he couldn't come home."

Her words helped me guide her, asking questions to clarify what was needed by her husband and her family, including how she could continue to best help her husband and manage the transition from home to a skilled care facility. During our meeting, we discussed the dynamics of the family and not only what was needed and possible for Mr. Nowak's physical, emotional, and end-of-life care but also what was needed by Mrs. Nowak to make this transition. It was time for Mr. Nowak to move into a facility that could care for his physical needs in a kind and competent way so that his wife and extended family could spend their energy providing him with emotional and spiritual support.

---

So many considerations (physical and emotional needs of the individual living with dementia and those who care for them) go into choosing a long-term care facility or nursing home, as can be seen from the discussion of the Nowak family. Once the decision to move has been made, the family remains a major contributor in care through advocacy, decision making, and emotional support for the individual residing in the nursing home.

## Choosing a Facility

Advocacy begins with choosing the best possible facility for the person with dementia. As hard as it is, know that there are resources to help you. Begin by deciding the major goals for your family. Examples are the approach to care, proximity for visiting, support for a particular need or behavior, and religious affiliation. Understanding the process can be daunting. If you like someone to "talk you through it," I highly recommend using the Eldercare Locator (800-677-1116), a public service that helps older adults and their families connect to services. If you prefer to search for service before speaking to anyone, visit adrc-tae.acl.gov. The Administration for Community Living (ACL), a service of the federal government, partners with several other administrative services (the Centers for Medicare and Medicaid Services and the Veterans Health Administration to name a few) to streamline discovery of services through a "No Wrong Door Systems," with the goal of aiding in the search for quality long-term care. Other potential resources to assist you in the process of finding care include the social workers and discharge planners from a home health agency (if you are currently working with one), the Area Agency on Aging, or the Center for Independent Living (ilru.org or 713-520-0232).

Once you've found the names of facilities that meet your initial criteria, wonderful guides and checklists to address the many other aspects in choosing a site have been created by the Centers for Medicare and Medicaid Services (www.medicare.gov/Pubs/pdf/02174 .pdf) and the National Consumer Voice for Long-term Care (http:// theconsumervoice.org/uploads/files/family-member/A-Consumer -Guide-To-Choosing-A-Nursing-Home.pdf). Of primary importance is that the facility meets Medicare and Medicaid standards. All facilities that receive subsidy from the federal government must be inspected. If they don't pass inspection, they are not certified. Ask any facility to provide you with their inspection report and certification. More in-depth information on choosing a long-term care facility can be found through each of these sources. Along with these checklists, it is important to remember during a visit to focus on what you see, smell, and feel. There will be individuals showing typical signs of advancing dementia, including crying out or asking for help, sleeping in chairs, and having bladder and bowel incontinence. Notice how the nurses and other staff respond to the residents and to each other. Focus on the attitude and approach of those who will be caring for your family member. This is where the questions on the checklist about staff turnover or mandatory overtime are important. If staff members are overworked, it will be difficult for them to provide compassionate care. If coworkers are kind to each other, they will be kind to residents as well.

Another approach in choosing a nursing home may be to contact the Long-Term Care Ombudsman through the National Ombudsman Resource Center, another service of the ACL. The ombudsman advocates for citizens and works to improve care and quality of life. This service is involved in visiting facilities to ensure residents' rights are protected, addressing concerns about finances, and assisting individuals in comparing nursing homes and providing information about complaints against facilities and how they were handled. A local ombudsman program can be found by calling 800-677-1116 or visiting ltcombudsman.org.

### After the Move

When your family member moves in, the advocacy continues. Visit and encourage others to visit as well. Interaction with the staff will help them get to know your family member better through stories or your interpretation of your family member's nonverbal communication. The staff at my mother's facility chatted with my mother about her grandchildren and me as they cared for her, making their interactions more meaningful and tender. They also learned how my mother used her eyebrows to communicate, like a maestro guides an orchestra. A certain lilt of the right brow definitely meant to back off and give her some time. When staff learned that, mouth care became much easier for all. If things are going well, compliments and celebrations are appreciated. When my daughter and I baked cookies together, we began to make double batches, one for home and one for my mom's place.

If things are not going as you'd like, it's a good idea to discuss the situation with the nursing director. If changes cannot be made or conditions do not improve, you will be there to observe and document what is happening. You may need to contact your local long-term care ombudsman to obtain guidance on your family member's rights and protective state and federal regulations.

## MODIFICATION OF PLANS AS SITUATION CHANGES

### Respite

---

#### BUILDING SUPPORT, UTILIZING RESOURCES
• *Sheila and Faye's Story* •

Sheila, a financial professional, was concerned about her mother, Faye. Sheila had taken a 1,000-mile trip to check on Faye after Faye was hospitalized after a fall. To her surprise and dismay, Sheila found evidence of the dementia Faye had been hiding during their frequent phone calls: outdated and little food, poor housekeeping, and overdue bills. It was evident that Faye could not remain on her own, and Sheila had Faye discharged from the hospital to a skilled nursing facility in Sheila's town. Unfortunately, Faye didn't "fit in" well there. Her cognitive ability was overall preserved, but her judgment was impaired. This "spotty" cognitive picture made living alone difficult.

Sheila talked of feeling inept in dealing with all her mother's care needs: stimulation, communication, visits, finances, including submitting for Title XIX benefits. She always felt guilty that she wasn't moving her mother into her own home. She described fear and confusion about how to deal with Faye's dementia and all that came with it, and how this was the most difficult time of year for Sheila's work schedule. I asked if there was anyone who could help. "I have two sisters, and there are six grandchildren." I said she might start looking there. Could the grandchildren help with stimulation, could someone do some research on Title XIX, could one sister become the communication expert? As we talked further, we learned that Sheila had connections with area geriatric care coordinators. "I don't know how I could ask them!" and she blushed a bit as she heard herself say this. I told her that many people forget to start building a support net or don't know how to. "Yes—I didn't even think to stop, look up and use my resources. I admit I was a bit embarrassed to and afraid my mother might object." This response is common.

---

There are challenges of caring for an individual with dementia. By the time someone has journeyed to the late stages of the disease, energy, and patience may be worn thin. Respite care provides breaks to aid in restoring energy or balance so that continuing to partner in the care of your family member can continue in a healthy way.

## Respite: Early, Often, and Regularly

Respite, in its best form, is called in early and often to provide shared care and to support the primary caregiver. It may take time to become comfortable sharing care for a family member because of guilt, finances, fear, or a host of other reasons. But when you do, the rewards are many. The individual with dementia is happier and healthier, as are those partnering in care because they are fresh, fulfilled, and balanced in many areas of their life. So, why don't people start exploring respite options? The most common answers I hear include "I'm overwhelmed," "I couldn't ask anyone else to do this," and "My mother (or other family member) would never allow anyone else to help." When respite is not sought until exhaustion, depression, physical illness, or abuse have set in, untangling the complications and finding respite become more complex. Early preparation and persistence in finding solutions will be well worth it.

Begin finding respite by outlining your family's goals and needs. When individuals with dementia are in late stages, respite is usually done in their place of residence. Common choices for short respite breaks are companionship or health aides. For more extended breaks, options include residential programs and caregiver training/respite camps.

Companionship services can be obtained through several organizations. Friends, family, faith-based community, college, and other nonprofit organizations may be contacted to inquire about volunteers who may visit for short periods in a home or assisted living setting to allow the primary caregiver to get away for a time. Some people seek this type of assistance only occasionally, but I recommend doing so on a regular basis. The regular break provides a time to enjoy some fun or nurturing activities, with the goal of returning to caregiving refreshed and renewed. The time also may be used to attend a caregiver support group to share ideas, frustrations, and resources. Other ideas for creative respite care may come from these groups.

## Suggestions for Finding Respite for Personal Care

Respite may also be needed for personal care in daily living activities, such as bathing, dressing, and toileting. In this case, a higher level of care and training may be required. An agency, if you are working with one, may take on the responsibility of selecting, vetting, and training the individual in personal care. If you hire someone independently, be sure to conduct in-depth interviews, be specific about what tasks will be required, request both work and personal references, and be sure to check on them. I recommend competency-based interview questions. If you know your family member may be reluctant to receive mouth care, ask interviewees for their experience in mouth care and how they handle someone who is resistant. Consider running a background check, especially if you plan to hire the individual for long term. Obtaining permission is required before doing so, and under the Fair Credit Reporting Act, you must use a Consumer Reporting Agency. Please check rules and regulations with an expert before proceeding. Using an established, reputable background checking service will avoid most issues, but if you have further concerns, consult an employment and labor law firm. Look for a company that is a member of the National Association of Professional Background Screeners (NAPBS); this means the company complies with all the current rules and laws about background checks and is monitored. Payroll and tax obligations can be outsourced to a service for household employees or local bookkeeping and accounting services could be used.

## Day Programs

Adult day programs can be a wonderful resource to bridge care to provide stimulation or personal care for the individual living with dementia and to provide respite or time to work for those providing primary care. Day programs can offer a host of services, including counseling and support (for the individual and family members), recreational and arts activities, nutrition, therapies (for any physical, speech, or occupational needs), behavioral management, personal care, and some medical services (such as medication administration or blood pressure checks). Many day programs are geared to those with early and mid-stage dementia, but some are able to accommodate those with more advanced disease. Visit the programs in your area and ask questions. Understand what type of care is offered and if it will fit the escalating needs that accompany progression of the disease. Also, make sure that the program fits your needs. Is it adaptable for progression of disease or problematic behaviors? What are the financial considerations? Is there adequate staff and equipment to assist with increasing demands for personal and incontinence care? Are staff members trained in dementia issues? How? Can staff evaluate for changes in function? Are staff members aware of nonverbal communication? Is transportation available, and can it accommodate a wheelchair if needed?

Day programs can be immensely important for stimulation and several care needs, but more direct, personal care is usually needed to make a day program work for an individual as dementia progresses. The staff will assist in understanding what can and cannot be accommodated by the particular program.

## HOSPICE

Hospice is a term used for both a palliative approach to care and a health care benefit. A palliative approach is care that focuses on the comfort and dignity of the individual in his or her final months of life and includes families and caregivers. The focus is usually on alleviating pain or other disturbing symptoms, while supporting living, rather than on a cure for the underlying condition. Because pain or discomfort can be physical, mental, spiritual, or existential, the hospice approach requires a team that includes those with expertise in medicine (physicians, nurses, and health aides), counseling (social workers, counselors, and clergy), and respite (volunteers, family). Medicare hospice benefits are used in only about 11 percent of hospice claims because of difficulty in predicting prognosis in those with dementia and lack of recognition by health care providers of the use of hospice in this chronic, although terminal, condition. The majority of those with dementia die in a long-term care facility (67%). In a 2015 report, end-of-life knowledge and practice is low for staff, although interest in attaining additional training by staff was high.

## CASE MANAGEMENT AND PAID CAREGIVERS

How do you find the help you need as you decide on places for your family member to live and the services you need to make those decisions come to reality? Case management workers and caregivers are the most common way to start. When I receive a call from family members or friends, I often direct them to their local social worker, who can direct them to the social support in their region and to an individual (or group of individuals) who knows how and where to find and delegate to other resources. Your physician's office may also be able to direct you to resources. Family and friends may give you recommendations as well.

Online resources can also be helpful. Many of the resources that help in finding skilled nursing care can also help in finding in-home care and coordination services. The Eldercare Locator Online Tool (www.eldercare.gov/Eldercare.NET/Public/Index.aspx), supported by the US Administration on Aging, Department of Health and Human Services, covers multiple topics from caregivers, in-home services, and legal assistance to home repair and modification. The Alzheimer's Association can help find services through their community resource finder (www.communityresourcefinder.org), which houses a database with Alzheimer's Association programs and events, housing options, care at home, medical services, and community services. Medicare supports an online tool to compare home health services (at www.medicare.gov/homehealthcompare /search.html), including a home health care checklist (www.medicare .gov/what-medicare- covers/home-health-care/Home%20Health %20Agency%20Checklist.pdf).

## Geriatric Case Managers

A geriatric case manager can help coordinate many of the issues that arise and choices that need to be made in dementia care. Geriatric case managers are health and human services specialists who act as advocates or coaches/problem solvers for older adults and their families. They have experience or expertise in nursing, gerontology, social work, and/or psychology. Case managers are relatively expensive but are expert in many of the issues of transitioning across places of care and in managing problem solving and negotiating paid care.

There are three certification organizations for case management: Commission for Case Managers, the National Academy of Certified Care Managers, and the National Association of Social Workers (have both a Certified Social Work Case Manager and an advanced certification). The case manager should also hold a certification in his or her own field of study (for example, nursing or social work). The services offered can be put together by an individual family, but if financial resources are available, obtaining such expertise can streamline many care decisions.

---
### POINTS TO REMEMBER
---

▶ Choosing the appropriate place of care in the later stages of dementia requires understanding and navigation of the complexities of personal, emotional, and financial resources.

▶ Supplemental care (either paid or unpaid) will ease the burden often experienced by primary caregivers.

▶ Hospice care is often not sought for those with dementia, partly due to the difficulty in predicting prognosis, partly due to physicians trained more in acute than in chronic care and partly due to ignorance that dementia is an appropriate hospice condition.

▶ Respite care can be done in the home or, at times, in an assisted living facility, a skilled nursing facility, or an inpatient hospice facility. Most respite care is an out-of-pocket expense with some exceptions. An extended break for the primary caregiver is not as common as help in the home on a regular basis for short breaks.

─────────────────── **ACTION PLAN** ───────────────────

▶ If possible, begin planning for progression of disease and transitions in care early on. Planning will allow for the best living situation for all involved. Short, frequent discussions with the individual living with dementia and/or family members are good first steps to begin mapping the best way forward.

▶ Find one hour this month to explore options for the next level of functional decline for your family member. Use the resources discussed previously in this chapter. Is the best use of your time finding respite, visiting an assisted living or day program, finding a social worker or case manager, or speaking with a financial adviser? Allot one hour each month for similar exploration.

─────────── **ADDITIONAL READING AND RESOURCES** ───────────

▶ www.medicare.gov/Pubs/pdf/02174.pdf

This 60-page, comprehensive document compiled by the Department of Health and Human Services Centers for Medicare and Medicaid, assists in choosing a nursing home or other long-term care facility. The document reviews long-term care options, how to pay for nursing home care, the rights of those living in nursing homes, and alternatives to nursing home care.

▶ www.payingforseniorcare.com/

This website is funded by referral fee from eldercare service providers. The site was founded in 2007 by an attorney specializing in estate planning and legal issues for older adults. It is comprehensive, free of ads, easy to navigate, and informative in understanding the cost of services and comparisons of the services.

## 7

# Changing Care Needs at the End of Life

As someone with dementia moves into the later stages of their disease, a number of adaptations are typically needed. Recognizing changing communication abilities is important to maximize understanding and minimize pain or frustration. Tips and tricks to assist or undertake personal care are reviewed. Strategies for avoiding falls that accompany changes in walking and suggestions for when to adopt a wheelchair or hospital bed come into play. Several practical suggestions are offered for changes in daily care options.

---

### ADAPTING TO THE NEED FOR INCREASED CARE
#### • The Kenny Family Story •

When my mother first moved to live near me, we cherished Sundays. I would share lunch with my mom at her place, chatting with others from her wing about the weather or songs. Afterward, my mom would climb into my car for our Sunday drive, an outing to a museum or just a kitchen table visit at my house. The kids would pop in for a quick chat and my mother's famous squealing hug. My husband read her whatever interesting articles he was enjoying while I puttered preparing dinner or sorting through bills. My mom would help with dinner, snapping the green beans or tearing lettuce. We gauged my mom's decline by the changes in Sundays. The stroll to the car evolved to an arm-in-arm escort, then a ride in a wheelchair, and finally, a complete lift into and out of the car. The visits with kids advanced from playful smiles and jokes to blank stares or even scowls at their noise. A nap on the couch substituted for the stories with my husband who now silently read near her as she slept. On the dinner menu, fresh salads with lettuce and chopped carrots changed to cooked spinach to avoid choking episodes.

Much changed during the late stages of my mother's decline. She communicated less, and more antics were needed to elicit a smile. She required far more rest; complete assistance with bathing, toileting, and mouth care; and modifications to her diet. She moved from walking quickly to shuffling tentatively, progressing to falls, and then an inability to walk. She spent most of her final months in bed. These changes required daily adaptation to allow for her best life possible.

---

## COMMUNICATING

Language has likely changed dramatically in your family member throughout the course of the disease. Early on, there were missed words or loss of train of thought. As the disease progressed, you probably noticed a lack of logical organization or less speech. In the final stages, there is often a further shift into reliance on nonverbal communication, such as facial expressions, vocalizations, or hand gestures. So, what can be done? I know that I continued to speak with my mother and imagined what she might be saying by looking at her face, putting some words to the emotions I was guessing at and then asking her if that was correct. For example, if I told her a story about the boys being rambunctious with their friends, she might scowl a bit. I would then ask, "You don't like it when the boys get in trouble?" If her face remained relatively flat, I would try again. "You probably had trouble with my brothers like that sometimes, right?" Her face would soften and she might close her eyes as if remembering. I felt this was a successful "moment" when we made a connection in her late stage of disease.

More often than not, I would simply sit with my mother and be. If she was awake, we used the time to put lotion on her hands and arms, talking about the creamy texture and enjoying the touch. Or we'd sit outside, and I would comment on the birds, flowers, or passersby while she sat in silence. Her calmness would be my sense that we were communicating well. The key to communication in the final stages of dementia is exploring options to find joy and comfort.

## Distressed Language or Vocalizations

When the communication seems disturbed, signaled by crying, moaning, or agitated vocalizations, consider triggers. Might there be hunger, fatigue, pain, boredom, or overstimulation? How do you decide? Trial and error. Guesswork. Knowing your family member. Look for signs and signals to assist in understanding whether fatigue or hunger is the cause of the unrest. My sister would keep notes and review them for clues, including phases of the moon, my mother's mood, time of day, and what type of rest or stimulation had occurred the day before. With my mother, an active day was best followed by a quieter day or she would become easily frustrated and angry. We learned, through trial and error, that a party or a doctor appointment should be followed by a low-key day with time for an extra nap or quiet time.

Pain is a common cause of disturbed communication. Assessing pain in individuals with advanced dementia can be difficult. A standardized scale, such as the Pain Assessment in Advanced Dementia Scale, can be very helpful. The scale ranks symptoms of breathing (normal, occasional labored/hyperventilation, noisy labored, or long periods of hyperventilation), negative speech or sounds (moaning, calling out, crying), facial expression (sad, frightened, or grimacing), tense body language (pacing, fidgeting, clenched fists, pulled into oneself, or pushing/striking out), and the inability to console or distract the individual from restlessness or crying. Scoring is easy; the higher the score, the more intense the distress. There is research evidence that the scale matches self-report in those with early cognitive decline and comparability between caregiver's impressions of pain in individuals with advanced dementia.

If pain is the cause of problems, nonpharmacologic strategies, such as warm soaks, ice packs, medicated rubs, gentle stretching, and massage, may supplement mild pain medications and stronger pain medications if necessary. Speak with your physician about treatment options. A trial of a stronger pain medication may be necessary, but you will need to advocate for your family member, because many physicians try to avoid stronger medications due to side effects, which include constipation, sedation, and the potential for addiction. Because your family member is in the end stages of a chronic but terminal disease and the goal is to provide comfort, a trial of these medications is likely warranted.

## DAILY CARE

Daily care becomes more and more the responsibility of the care partner as dementia progresses. The individual living with dementia may lose the ability to perform the multistep tasks required to perform daily care and fear, vulnerability, and embarrassment may remain. Care partners, as hard as it is to believe, need to be even more patient and adaptable. As has been required throughout the disease progression, flexibility and an individual approach are necessary. When a process is not working, try new approaches or ask others for suggestions. Support groups, online chat rooms, other family members, and health care providers can all be helpful.

### Bathing

One of the most common challenges is resistance to showering or bathing. Family members report concern when their family member will not willingly participate in a bath or cleaning up. As with many challenging behaviors or situations, the first approach is to gather information and consider all angles. Does there need to be a bath at all? Many families tell me, "My father won't shower every day" when the need for a full bath may not be necessary and just washing face, hands, feet, underarms, and the genital area may be enough.

If the individual physically resists, yells, or curses or shows signs of fear such as crying, shaking, or withdrawing, are there any clues to determine the reason? With some care, issues of modesty, temperature, or lack of control can be addressed.

## BATHING WITH TENDERNESS AND DIGNITY
### • Janet and Lillian's Story •

Janet, a kind, tender nursing aid, transferred Lillian from her wheelchair to a shower chair and rolled her into the warm room. As Janet prepared the soap, washcloth, and warm towels, she spoke and sang softly with Lillian. Janet prepared the room with warm air and prewarmed the shower. The scent of lavender wafted around the lowered lights and soft music. The institutional bathroom took on the mood and feel of a luxury spa. Once the air was warm, Janet removed Lillian's shoes and socks and placed her feet in a warm, scented tub to soak. Janet placed a warm towel on Lillian's shoulders and began a gentle massage. All the while, Janet softly murmured, telling Lillian what was coming next and obtaining Lillian's nonverbal assent.

Janet faced Lillian and asked her if they could change into a shower top. Janet replaced Lillian's blouse and bra with a short terrycloth robe and placed another warmed towel on Lillian's chest. Lillian's face and body were very relaxed. Janet kneeled in front of Lillian, washed her feet and then tugged on rubber-bottomed slippers. Janet removed Lillian's pants and covered her waist and legs with a towel. Using a handheld showerhead, Janet then washed Lillian's hair, always keeping an eye on Lillian for signs of distress and placing a clean, warm towel on Lillian's shoulder to keep water from her eyes. Janet then washed Lillian's arms, chest, and back, being careful to keep Lillian covered at all times. Janet told me since she had learned to keep Lillian covered with warm towels, Lillian had stopped fighting bath time. After Lillian's upper body was cleaned, the wet towels were replaced with warm dry towels. Janet then cleaned Lillian's backside and legs and examined the area for any irritation or skin issues. Finally, Janet dried Lillian carefully, protecting her tender skin by always using a patting motion to avoid friction from rubbing.

---

The bathing process that Janet used for Lillian was effective for several reasons. A calm and relaxed atmosphere was created before the actual bathing began. The room temperature was warmed. Lillian's attitude was considered. Her family and staff had learned that maintaining Lillian's modesty was paramount to her agreeable participation. Janet focused on safety with nonskid slippers and dried areas soon after washing to avoid Lillian becoming chilled. Janet involved Lillian throughout the process, holding towels and washcloths and encouraging singing.

Others may need baths or handheld shower attachments with a soft, gentle flow, because showering water, whether due to sound or perceived sting, is disturbing to many individuals living with dementia. Often, baths may need to be done in bed or in a chair. The procedures for a bed or chair bath are relatively straightforward: protect the bed or chair with thick bath towels. Make sure the room is warm enough and the individual being bathed is covered for warmth and modesty. The bath is usually done on one side of the body and then the other, washing, rinsing, and drying one section of the body at a time (using different washcloths and towels for each area), working from head to arms/chest/abdomen and then to the legs and genitals. Soap should be rinsed thoroughly to avoid its drying properties on aging skin. Skin should be dried using a patting motion; rubbing results in friction that may tear or otherwise damage skin. Many of my patients' families have used a home health agency to train them in strategies for bathing. The training helps with so many issues, including positioning and technique to avoid injury for the care partner, alleviating anxiety of performing a task that is new, and learning coping strategies to lessen the discomfort and embarrassment of caring for another person's body. More suggestions and videos are also available online. The Alzheimer's Association has a caregiver tip sheet for bathing (https://www.alz.org/cacentral/documents/Dementia_Care_32 -_The_Battle_of_the_Bathing.pdf). If bed baths are required, it is likely time for a hospital bed to assist the caregiver in providing care.

As dementia progresses, urinary and/or fecal incontinence may increase the need for bathing and thorough cleaning. Using large disposable washcloths or developing a system of using a series of damp washcloths can assist in cleaning throughout the day or night when a complete bath is not needed. If skin shows signs of redness, irritation, rashes or breakdown, a more comprehensive approach is necessary (see discussion on incontinence).

## Dressing

In the late stages of dementia, the caregiver needs to dress the individual living with dementia. The specific clothing may make dressing easier and/or more comfortable. Continue to query your family member for style or color choices to retain as much independence as possible. Concentrating on materials your family member enjoys can provide sensory enjoyment. My mother loved the feel of velvet, so velour was a nice choice for her. Ease of washing the clothing is also a consideration. Many individuals living with dementia do not enjoy having clothes pulled over their heads, so selecting shirts, sweaters, and jackets that have front closures is helpful. Layering clothes can help individuals remain neither too hot nor cold. In intimate apparel, if a bra is necessary for support and comfort, a front closing bra is much easier to handle. Boxer shorts are easier to don than tighter fitting underwear for men, although incontinence briefs are commonly needed. Pants with elasticized waistbands are easier to pull on than those with a button and zipper; many are "camouflaged" with a zipper appearance. Specialty clothes are available that have easy snap or hook-and-loop closures in the back or side snaps (on pants) with a wide opening for ease with toileting.

As with other personal care, courtesies such as privacy, room temperature, and adequate time should be thought out and planned before beginning any procedure. Special considerations include the potential need for a supportive chair during dressing as the individual may not be capable of maintaining his or her balance while sitting up on a bed.

## Mouth Care

Care of the mouth is often neglected. Understanding basic mouth care techniques and mastering strategies to care for individuals living with cognitive impairment has resulted in better overall care and fewer episodes of pneumonia, a common consequence of poor oral health. The University of North Carolina at Chapel Hill developed and studied a program called Mouth Care Without a Battle. An excellent worksheet that reviews the techniques established to work can be found online at http://files.www.mouthcarewithoutabattle .org/about-mouth-care/Mouth_Care_Basics_Worksheet.pdf. The worksheet has stepwise instructions for providing care and a product list (http://files.www.mouthcarewithoutabattle.org/ce-forms /Product_Selection_Flowsheet.pdf).

The procedures include cleaning the preparation/work area with a sanitizing cloth, setting up the needed equipment, washing your hands and donning nonlatex gloves, dipping the toothbrush in the cleaning paste or solution, and then cleaning each tooth with a jiggle at the gumline, followed by a rotary motion and then downward (or upward) sweeping motion to move plaque away from the gumline. Clean the toothbrush periodically with a clean gauze square, and reapply cleaning paste or solution. Once the brushing is completed, use an interdental brush to floss each tooth in a systematic fashion. Clean the tongue with a tongue-cleaner, either the back of a toothbrush designed for this purpose or a cotton swab wrapped in gauze that has been dipped in cleaning solution. Finally, use a cotton-tipped applicator to place a thin layer of fluoride rinse on each tooth, beginning on the outer surface. Clean the toothbrush and interdental brush after with an antibacterial rinse and dry after each use. Replace the toothbrush and interdental cleaners at least every three months or when wear is evident.

The person-centered approach is helpful in oral care. Provide verbal cues of what you will be doing and physical cues such as touching the lip with a brush. Allow the individual to rest as needed. Consistency increases success in oral care, so it is important for this to be a daily procedure. If there are resistive behaviors, several strategies may be used to improve success. As with all care, personalizing the care is paramount. Be curious about what may be causing the refusal (fear, pain, fatigue) and then address the issue or try redirecting with songs and conversation. Several tips specific to mouth care, including gently rubbing the cheek to relax jaw muscles, or jiggling the toothbrush if the person is biting on it and asking them to open their mouth, are outlined in the following handout: http://files.www .mouthcarewithoutabattle.org/best-practices/MCWB_Behavior _Strategies.pdf.

## Eating

*Adapting the Meal Experience*

In chapter 5, we discussed how eating may be modified to avoid prolonging dying with dementia. While eating may still be enjoyable and social, consider simplifying the food choices. During my mother's middle stages of dementia, she became overwhelmed by all the menu selections in a restaurant, but if my sister asked if she'd like chicken or fish, my mother would choose one easily. My sister would then order for her. I used a similar technique when I saw that my mother seemed overwhelmed by a full plate of food offered all at once. I placed each food item separately on a smaller plate and offered her one at a time. First, she would eat the peas and carrots, then the chicken (which I cut for her while she was eating the vegetables), and finally the mashed potatoes. Some adaptive utensils and plates may maintain independence longer; for example, utensils with larger, rubber handles allow for easier grasping of food, and plates with rimmed edges can help when scooping up food. Occupational therapists can provide specific guidance on adaptive solutions to increase independence with eating. Occupational therapists may be available through your assisted living facility or can be found through a home nursing service or local hospital.

### Appetite and Taste

Appetite and taste will change. Remember to adapt your expectations of your family member's nutritional needs as his or her life changes. Caloric needs are less because of lower activity levels and as the end of life approaches. Tastes change with dementia and sweeter foods are often preferred. My mother lived on ice cream for several months.

### Swallowing

As swallowing becomes more difficult, changing food to a pureed consistency may help avoid difficulty with chewing and choking. This change signifies that the swallowing mechanism is affected. The time will come when the ability to move food or drink from the front of the mouth to the back and then coordinate the swallowing motion is lost. Choking, food remaining in the mouth (called pocketing), or a thick voice indicate that this is occurring. Pneumonia may develop as food is no longer effectively swallowed but instead aspirated into the lungs. Even saliva is no longer swallowed and leads to aspiration. This is another reason why placement of a feeding tube will not avoid pneumonia. Saliva is formed continually, in the absence of food and regardless of a feeding tube.

## Toileting

Incontinence, or the involuntary loss of urine or stool, is likely well known to a care partner by the end of the journey with dementia. The lack of recognition of the signals from the body to the brain that urine or stool is being passed, recognizing the steps in undressing, or understanding where the bathroom is or its purpose were likely lost in the earlier stages of dementia.

*Timed Voiding*

Incontinence can be approached with timed, prompted voiding in the late stages of dementia. Timed, prompted voiding is a type of habit training. It involves setting a schedule for urinating (such as every two hours or another time interval based on personal need) with the goal of decreasing accidents and wet or soiled clothing. Although timed, prompted voiding will not avoid all accidents, it can decrease their number. Some caregivers use the top of the even (or odd) hours to remind them to check for accidents, and some use a watch alarm as a reminder.

*Modifiable Triggers for Incontinence: Constipation, Caffeine, Medications*

One of the leading causes of reversible overactive bladder is constipation because when the colon is full, it puts pressure on the bladder. Constipation can be addressed by increasing fiber in the diet and maintaining good hydration. Eating fruits that are high in water content may be a way to increase hydration. A mixture of applesauce, bran flakes, and prune juice (equal parts) given daily (2–4 tablespoons) is a natural way to increase fiber. This mixture has been used by many of my patients with excellent results, avoiding the roller coaster of constipation and diarrhea that may accompany taking stool softeners and laxatives. If a natural approach is not effective, please consult your health care provider for advice on next steps.

Another trigger for overactive bladder is caffeinated drinks and some medications. Use of herbal teas, decaffeinated coffee, or just warm water may avoid some of the stimulation to the bladder from caffeine. Diuretics are commonly used medications, and the timing of their administration can be coordinated with a toileting schedule or other event. For example, voiding usually needs to occur an hour or two after a diuretic is given, so toileting should be more frequent during this time. If an outing is planned, administration of the diuretic may be timed for after the individual is home. I have had many patients or family members remain home in the morning, missing enjoyable activities, trapped by the need to be near a toilet. They are relieved to know they can delay administration of the diuretic until lunch time so they can accommodate other activities without endangering their health.

*Stigma: Gentle Emotions*
Incontinence can be disturbing to the individual and the care partner because of the social stigma. Many of my patients' families find that incontinence is the hardest of the caregiving needs, due to embarrassment of caring for the genital area of a spouse or parent. Many family members, when fatigued, have reported they think their family member has an accident "on purpose." Be gentle with your thoughts and feelings. It is important to assist someone with incontinence as soon as possible to decrease the risk of infection or skin breakdown. If you need a few minutes to catch your breath and calm your emotions, take that time so you can continue to provide the intimate care without becoming impatient or angry. Most find a straightforward, unembarrassed attitude helps with approach to the care.

*Incontinence Products*
Incontinence products such as adult briefs and bed pads are commonly used to help manage accidental wetting and soiling. Be sure to use incontinence pads and briefs that are designed to wick away moisture, because all risks for skin breakdown increase dramatically in a moist environment. Pressure ulcers occur in up to 24 percent of individuals in long-term care and 17 percent of individuals at home (see information on skin integrity and pressure ulcer prevention and approach). Moist washcloths can help keep skin clean and dry when used at times of toileting or brief changes. Incontinence-associated dermatitis, which is inflammation of the skin that occurs when urine or stool comes in contact with skin in the genital or anal area, results in rashes, irritation, pain, and skin breakdown. The National Pressure Ulcer Advisory Panel and European Pressure Ulcer Advisory Panel recommend a protective cream or ointment and disposable barrier wipes that provide cleaning, moisturizing, and a barrier cream to protect the skin. Many families buy multiple white, inexpensive

washcloths to be used with a pH neutral soap (some soaps cause an alkaline environment that is not natural) for incontinence care and do a load of laundry each night or two, placing the washcloths and towels in the dryer as they go off to bed. Others use disposable wash-cloths and towelettes. Special "barrier wipes" that clean, moisturize, and spread a protective barrier cream in one cloth are another op-tion. In a study of a complete comprehensive pressure ulcer preven-tion program that included the use of barrier wipes, pressure ulcers decreased dramatically. Incontinence-associated dermatitis occurs in about 25 percent of those with incontinence. In another study, barrier wipes were superior to the washcloth and a pH neutral soap, decreasing the rate of dermatitis from 27 percent to 8 percent. Both approaches work well, but the key to maintaining skin integrity is keeping the perineal area clean and dry.

## Skin Changes and Care

Many skin changes are seen with aging and often with situations that accompany dementia such as poor food and fluid intake. Skin protects us from the environment, regulates body temperature, and carries the receptors for touch, pain, and pressure. Skin changes are affected by genetics (light, fair-haired individuals will show more changes from sun damage than those with darker pigment, for ex-ample), nutrition, and other ongoing conditions.

Poor food and fluid intake may be expected in dementia and ac-centuates thinning of the skin that accompanies age. Aging skin also loses its strength and elasticity and produces less oil, which leads to a higher risk of tearing and dryness. In turn, dryness may lead to itchiness. It is important to minimize itching by moisturizing the skin with lotions and limiting use of soaps that can change the pH of the skin. Cleansers that maintain a neutral pH may be a better choice.

The subcutaneous fat layer, which is a layer of fat under the skin, provides insulation and padding. This layer also thins, again increas-ing risk of skin tearing and the individual feeling cold. When layering clothing to combat the sense of cold, the skin microenvironment may be altered in certain areas such as the perineum. This, too, leads to increased risk of pressure ulcers.

In addition to so many other losses, the loss of movement accompanies late-stage dementia. Your family member may remain in bed or a chair and not move or even change position enough to allow circulation to the areas of skin under pressure. This lack of movement is yet another risk for pressure ulcers.

## PREVENTION OF PRESSURE ULCERS

Pressure ulcers are best prevented by first assessing for risk factors and modifying those that can be changed.

### Change of Position

This is one of the most crucial recommendations to prevent pressure ulcers and should occur every two hours. Changing the position of the body allows for improved circulation to the compressed area. The area needs to be clean and dry, and the sheets or other surface should not have folds. This is easier said than done, but it is always helpful to check and try to smooth any folds that are present. An individual may have a preferred place to rest and will move right back to the area after being moved off. Bony areas or bony protrusions will be at risk of skin breakdown. Pillows or a pad can be used to protect those areas (or preferred positions) around the hips, buttocks, heels, elbows, and ears. Cushioning devices positioned to keep someone lying on his or her side can help prevent pressure on bony prominences. The goal is to offload pressure from high-risk areas. Once the individual has been repositioned, it is important to check that the pressure has been offloaded. This may seem daunting—how can someone at home learn all these tricks? A session with a pressure ulcer specialist from a local visiting nurse company will help you to learn these techniques.

## Friction and Reducing Shear

Sliding motion against sheets creates shear, or friction. Those who require moderate to maximum assistance in moving in a bed or chair are at high risk. Agitated activity in bed is another cause for shear forces to affect the skin. Lying with the head elevated above 30 degrees in bed or in a slouched position in a chair also puts shear forces on the lower back / sacral area.

## Moisture

Skin that is often or always moist, due to sweating or incontinence, is at high risk of breakdown. All the other factors, including immobility, reduced sense of pain (so that a sore or pressure is not felt and avoided or moved away from), or poor nutrition, become additive when they occur in a moist skin environment. Skin that is kept clean and moisturized is less likely to develop pressure ulcers. Drying soaps should be avoided.

## Nutrition

As mentioned earlier, poor food and fluid intake are expected with advancing dementia. Ensuring nutritional support will help in both wound healing and preventing skin breakdown.

## ADDITIONAL PRESSURE ULCER CONCERNS

At the end of life, other concerns may supersede the prevention of pressure ulcers. The National Pressure Ulcer Advisory Panel has published a thoughtful article that assists in balancing, understanding, and personalizing the issues that likely may need modification at the end of life. For example, although frequent turning is needed when someone is sleeping up to 20 hours per day or some other form of nutritional support may be considered, goals of care may shift to comfort rather than pressure ulcer treatment and management as the end of life care is prioritized. Set treatment goals based on quality of life, not necessarily on healing the ulcer or wound because this may not be possible, depending on the underlying cause and the person's nutritional status.

Pressure ulcers are often found after a stay in the hospital. Pressure ulcers acquired in the hospital are the fourth leading cause of preventable medical error in the United States. Standardized scales are available to help predict who is at high risk of pressure ulcer development. These scales assess mobility, activity, sensory perception, nutrition, moisture, and sheer/friction force. The Braden Scale is most widely used. The skin needs to be inspected daily, from head to toe, for areas at risk or areas of breakdown, at the time of turning, bathing, or dressing.

If a pressure ulcer develops in someone who is not able to communicate well, the individual is very likely experiencing pain. Pain is reported in nearly all pressure ulcers. Therefore, pain should be presumed, and the individual premedicated 20–30 minutes before changing his or her dressings or position.

If a pressure ulcer does develop, the assistance of a wound specialist from a nursing or hospice agency should be considered. The multiple approaches need to be individualized, and the expertise of a specialist can minimize discomfort and improve the quality of life of the individual and the family.

## CHANGES IN MOBILITY AND THE NEED FOR LIFTING

As the ability to walk deteriorates, falls will increase and, ultimately, most individuals living with dementia are confined to a chair and a bed. Procedures to manage toileting, incontinence, perineal rashes, bathing, dressing, and feeding can all be adapted for those who are unable to leave their chair or bed. The biggest change that accompanies the loss of mobility is the need for the caregiver to lift the family member to aid in transfers and care.

In a small study of informal caregivers, one in three was injured from lifting or caring for their dependent family member. Back injuries were the most common, accounting for more than half of the injuries. One quarter of the reported injuries resulted in caregivers no longer being able to care for their family member. Most caregivers had received only sporadic, informal instruction and most felt training would have been useful.

Safe handling, transferring, and lifting requires skills and an awareness of the caregiver's limitations. If the caregiver is frail or has health issues, lifting or transferring another person may not be feasible.

---

### LEARNING PHYSICAL LIMITS IN TRANSFERRING
#### • *The Quincys' Story* •

Mr. and Mrs. Quincy were married 62 years. They did everything together, so it was no surprise when Mrs. Quincy wanted to care for Mr. Quincy at home as his function declined from complications of dementia. As Mr. Quincy entered the late stages of dementia, his gait became more and more unsteady, and he started to have falls. Mrs. Quincy stayed in close proximity to Mr. Quincy, to aid him in getting to the bathroom if he felt a sudden urge. She was also losing sleep, because at times he would bolt out of bed to try to get to the bathroom. She had tried a timed voiding schedule, but Mr. Quincy's erratic bolting continued. Mr. Quincy was twice the size of Mrs. Quincy, so when he lost his balance, she had a difficult time steadying him.

Family, friends, and I had all cautioned Mrs. Quincy that Mr. Quincy was too large for her to handle physically by herself, but she insisted she could manage. As she slept less and became fatigued, she began falling with Mr. Quincy. Finally, one sad day, I received a call at home. "Dr. Kenny, I'm on the floor with Norm, and we can't get up. I can't move my leg." I called the ambulance and the Quincys' daughter to meet us at the hospital. Mrs. Quincy had broken her hip. Mr. Quincy went home with his daughter, and the process to have him cared for in a long-term care facility was begun.

---

The Quincys' story is not unusual, but the injury might have been prevented if Mrs. Quincy had acknowledged her growing fatigue and Mr. Quincy's increased dependence as his disease progressed. Training in proper lifting strategies can help, but it is critical to understand the limits of a single person to do all the lifting for another, especially in the case of unexpected toileting needs or when behavior issues make transfers difficult and falls highly unpredictable. Also, if the body size differences are too great, assistance from only one person may not be possible.

## LEARNING TO LIFT

Injury may occur from improper body mechanics or repeated lifts when the muscles are fatigued. Both of these situations are common when caring for a physically dependent family member.

### Body Mechanics

The key to preventing injury is to keep your body in the proper alignment. The body structure is based on bones, joints, and the muscle and tendons that move the bone and joints. The spine is the most likely to be injured. The spine is a tower of bones that are held by a thin series of muscles, much like guidewires from the top to the bottom of the tower. The muscles in the spine are small compared with the muscles of the legs. This is why the primary rule is to lift with your legs, not your back.

## How to Lift

When lifting, keep your back straight. Do not bend from the waist. The muscles of your back are meant to keep your spine upright, not to lift heavy loads. If your back is rounded, the muscles are not aligned to hold your spine and your head will jut out, rather than being held over your shoulder, which strains your neck muscles. The stress becomes greater when you then add more weight by lifting. Also be sure to hold your stomach firm. Holding your stomach muscles in creates pressure in your abdominal cavity that helps to support your lower back. Note that holding your stomach in does not mean holding your breath. You should continue to breathe normally while lifting, and it is recommended you exhale during a lift to ensure that you are not holding your breath. A stance that will provide balance and support for lifting is one in which you keep your feet shoulder width apart, with one foot slightly in front of the other. This wide base of support allows movements side to side and forward and back without losing your balance. For the lift itself, you should bend at the knees, staying close to the person (or object), while keeping your back straight and aligned. Use your powerful hip and leg muscles for the actual lift. By keeping the person close to your body, you will have better control in keeping their weight centered over your legs, rather than straining your back muscles. The use of a gait belt (a specialized belt worn securely and snugly around the waist of the individual who needs assistance with lifting and transferring) provides a way to support the individual, assist if balance is lost, or provide a way to safely lower the person to the bed or floor. Use of the belt should be learned from a physical or occupational therapist.

I'm often asked if back supports or braces are helpful. Back supports should be used to remind you of proper body mechanics, not as a true support. They do not add strength and will not prevent an improper lift. Helpful ideas include planning ahead, keeping one surface close to another (such as the wheelchair and bed), and using a hospital bed so that the bed can be raised to a height to assist in care or lifts. Face squarely the person you are assisting, and do not twist the trunk of your body to make a move. Always turn your feet and encourage your family member to do the same during a transfer.

To lift or boost someone in bed, if possible ask your family member to assist by bending his or her knees and pushing for you on the count of three. If the individual cannot follow directions, be sure to use an additional sheet or pad to lift, thereby minimizing the shearing or sliding of the skin on the bedsheets. Continue to protect your back during a boost by placing one knee on the bed to simulate the staggered foot stance and wide base of support described previously. Keep the person close to your body to minimize bending your back and using your weaker back muscles. Always keep your back straight. If using a hospital bed, raise the bed to your waist level to avoid leaning at the waist. Do not have your family member hold you around the neck because this will put unnecessary strain on your neck.

Lifting equipment, such as a Hoyer, Sara, or Vera lift, should be used only after training from a specialist such as a nurse or physical therapist. The use of mechanical devices to aid in lifting is a specific technique that requires consultation with a specialist.

——————————————  POINTS TO REMEMBER  ——————————————

▶ Communication may shift to more nonverbal communication. Watch your family member's facial expressions and emotional state to guide your actions and discussions.

▶ Signs and symptoms of pain are relatively standard and include breathing (normal, occasional labored/hyperventilation; noisy labored, or long periods of hyperventilation), negative speech or sounds (moaning, calling out, crying), facial expression (sad, frightened, or grimacing), tense body language (pacing, fidgeting, clenched fists, pulled into oneself or pushing/striking out), and the inability to console or distract the individual from restlessness or crying.

▶ Daily care needs should be modified to provide support in a personalized way as independence is lost. Bathing, dressing, toileting, and eating will require more direct support. Baths may need to be done in bed, clothing choices may need modification so that another can help, and scheduled toileting may be needed, along with frequent changes of incontinence pads or briefs with cleaning of the area.

▶ Better health outcomes and quality of life have been observed with good oral care. Mouth Care Without a Battle is a proven method to train yourself or family members in how to assist in oral care.

▶ Modifying the consistency of food, adding sweetness to food, and increasing liquids (over solid food intake) are common early strategies to use as appetite and adeptness at self-feeding is lost. When swallowing becomes difficult and choking starts to occur, review the goals of care to prepare for the final phase of life, adjust to the weight loss, and support quality experiences focused less on food.

▶ Minimize incontinent episodes by treating constipation, modifying timing of medications, minimizing substances that stimulate the bladder, and attempting a timed voiding schedule.

▶ When incontinence occurs, minimize the time urine or stool is in contact with skin to optimize skin care and avoid incontinence-associated dermatitis or pressure ulcers.

▶ Pressure ulcers are best prevented by changing positions, minimizing shearing forces on the skin, controlling moisture (incontinence and sweat), and providing good nutrition. Obviously, all these conditions cannot be maximized when the focus shifts to end-of-life care. At that point, personal choices and comfort on positioning and nutrition must be balanced with adequate pain control and local skin care.

▶ As mobility becomes more limited and an individual transitions to increased time in a chair or a bed, proper lifting techniques will prevent injury to both the caregiver and family member. The first tenet is to understand the physical limits to lifting, and if the situation is unsafe, assistance should be sought.

▶ Proper lifting techniques should be studied and practiced with every lift.

───────────────────  ACTION PLAN  ───────────────────

▶ To aid in nonverbal communication, journal to track what certain expressions or behaviors may signal fatigue, hunger, or joy.

▶ Journal or track symptoms that are consistent with pain such as labored breathing, negative speech or sounds, tense body language, restlessness, and crying. Then track what actions make it better or worse, including but not limited to food, quiet, stimulation, pain reliever, warm soaks, or rest.

▶ If any aspects of personal care (bathing, dressing, toileting, mouth care, incontinence care) are difficult or daunting, contact a local health care agency to provide training in care.

▶ Prevent pressure ulcers by understanding their cause and actions that can help to prevent them: change positions, avoid shearing forces, keep the area dry, and support good nutrition.

▶ Practice proper lifting with every lift: keep your back straight, lift with your legs, hold in your stomach, use a staggered, shoulder-width stance, and stay close to the person being lifted.

───────── ADDITIONAL READING AND RESOURCES ─────────

Few books are available to guide you on daily care. Many websites have wonderful resources and information.

▶ The Alzheimer's Association (alz.org)

This website has a host of material. A Caregiver Center links to daily care strategies for daily plans, activities, communication, food and eating, music and art, and personal care issues, such as incontinence, bathing, dressing, grooming, and dental care.

▶ Alzheimer's Foundation of America (Alzfdn.org)

This website, founded in 2002 with a mission to provide optimal care and services to individuals living with Alzheimer disease and related dementias, has a caregiving resources section that supplies fact sheets and information on fall prevention, incontinence, eating tips, understanding behaviors as a form of communication, and more.

▶ The Family Caregiver Alliance (www.caregiver.org)

Information on this website is plentiful, including a comprehensive list of resources for classes, videos, fact sheets, webinars, and more.

# 8

# Changing Needs for the Caregiver/Partner at the End of Life

The statistics on caregiving, or care partnering, are staggering. Approximately 45 million US adults care for another adult person, and nearly all (83%) comes from family, friends, or unpaid caregivers. This care is, without a doubt, accompanied by much cost in terms of time, money, and emotions. Unpaid caregiving takes hours of time— hours of time that now are not available for other family members or to work. And what happens when the caregiving needs continue to increase as dementia progresses toward the end of life?

---

### KNOWING WHEN IT'S TIME TO GET HELP
#### • The Kenny Family Story •

I cried. Every night. On my way home, sometimes the crying started before I even left the lobby of the assisted living facility. Quietly, if my kids were with me. More openly if alone with the car windows down, gulping in big mouthfuls of air as I released my stress and sadness. The woman in the mirror had become unrecognizable. I was haggard, with bloodshot eyes, my mouth in a perpetual frown or scowl. I was doing too much and had missed the warning signs along the way—and there had been many. A gentle suggestion from my husband that I might be adding too many activities would be met with a snappish, "What have I missed?" My kids would sigh when I phoned that dinner was in the crockpot but that I would be home "in a bit." Work colleagues would offer a cup of coffee after they saw me nodding off at conferences or dragging in late for a meeting. I knew it was bad when I couldn't remember the last time I had laughed—and normally I laugh a lot! I laugh when I'm happy, embarrassed, guilty, nervous, or frustrated, but not when I'm exhausted or sad. And I was definitely exhausted and sad.

All self-help books remind us to *first* take care of ourselves in order to have something to give; flight attendants start each flight advising passengers to put on their own oxygen mask before helping others. As a caregiver, I needed help—in many ways. I took inventory and first figured out what I needed: time, support, exercise, calm, and fun. I figured out what my family needed: help with homework and some family fun. And I figured out what my mother needed: focused attention in the evenings. I learned to ask for help, pay for help, and barter for help. I started using short blocks of time (10–20 minutes) in very different ways to acquire what I needed to care for myself while I cared for my mother. I started slowly but made sure I made changes each week. First, I found a fabulous woman to visit and care for my mother four nights per week. It took time and energy to find her, but it was time well spent. If I had done only one thing, it would have been this. It freed me up to spend time with my kids, go on my usual monthly outing with girlfriends, finish my work, and get to bed on time more often than not. I had the energy to start exercising with my mom. We did silly chair aerobics and chair yoga from videos and, although she didn't always participate, at least it entertained her. I found a good therapist and began to meditate daily, to help with the crying and the grief and to cultivate the calm I craved.

---

## THE SCOPE OF IMPACT OF CAREGIVING

A comprehensive 2016 report by the Alzheimer's Association estimates that those living with dementia receive 18 *billion* hours of unpaid assistance annually. Ninety-two percent of individuals living in the community with dementia rely on at least one other person to assist them, and 30 percent rely on three or more caregivers. The Alzheimer's Association report goes on to describe who is delivering this care. Most caregivers (66%) live in the same house with the individual with dementia. Most individuals who report having the most responsibility for care are women (66%), often daughters (33%), with a college degree or greater (40%) but who have a household income of $50,000 or less. The time spent in caregiving disproportionately falls to women, putting in more hours per week in care than men. Finally, nearly one-quarter of those providing care to someone with Alzheimer or related dementia were also providing care to children younger than 18 years old, that is, the "sandwich generation" caregiver.

---

### BEING A "SANDWICH GENERATION" CAREGIVER
#### • *June's Story* •

June was a happy, funny woman who also could turn stern and steely-eyed in a flash if she felt her three children or her mother's well-being was being jeopardized. They all lived together, sharing lots of emotional and mutual support. June and I were friends via volunteer work. At volunteer events, she would tell me about her mother's memory and cognitive loss and how everyone in the family was coping. June's mother helped her with after-school child care by taking the kids to after-school activities and check-ups and by starting the family dinner. Most important to June, her mom kept the squabbling kids from getting into real trouble until June made it home from work.

Fast-forward three years. Mrs. Yates forgot to pick up the kids on one occasion. She was becoming easily irritated by the kids' noise, and dinner preparation was becoming less consistent. June knew more support was needed. Their first step was to have the oldest daughter, now 15, begin to assist her grandmother with schedules and meal prep. But June and Mrs. Yates were looking for more advice. The biggest issue was how to get the household to accommodate *everyone*. The stresses of Mrs. Yates's changes were affecting every family member. While June was a very positive and proactive caregiver, her needs were lost in the middle between the needs of her children and her mother. June had stopped exercising, was eating more and gaining weight, and had stopped dating.

In June's words, the stress was caused by the combination of her mother's escalating care needs, her mother's resistance to relinquishing her role in caring for the kids, June's own sadness at her mother's continued decline, and that it had all been going on for a few years.

During a recent visit with June and her mother, June courageously spoke up. She wanted to talk with me and her mom about the need to either change the family's living situation or explore strategies to help Mrs. Yates stay home. June had always honored her mom's opinions, even with her mother's reduced decision-making capabilities and memory loss. June reported that her mom became more agitated and restless when she was left in the morning and would call June repeatedly, leaving anxious messages. Mrs. Yates had more recently started leaving the house and had become lost on several occasions, walking for hours before finding the school or the police station. Mrs. Yates remembered only one of these episodes and felt she was safe to stay home. June wanted to learn about day programs or assisted living, which was upsetting to her mom. We began the difficult conversation.

Mrs. Yates died in her sleep about a week later, probably from a stroke. June was concerned that the conversation about changing living situations had contributed to, or even caused, her mother's death. We discussed the challenges of adjusting care in the late stages of her mother's dementia and that changes were needed for the entire family. June had many mixed emotions. She admitted relief that her mom wouldn't have to move but expressed regret that she didn't have the resources to more completely meet her mom's needs and guilt that the conversation and stress about need for change may have contributed to her mom's stroke. Although there is no way to know if there was any actual basis for June's concern, these were her true emotions.

# IMPACT OF CAREGIVING AND STRATEGIES TO HELP

## Caregiving Impact on Physical Health

### RECOGNIZING THE STRESS AND POTENTIAL HEALTH CONSEQUENCES OF CAREGIVING

• *The Murrays* •

It was the first day of clinic for Dr. Wong, a new trainee in geriatric medicine. She was quiet and polite. As I was orienting her to the flow of clinic and clinic procedures, Mr. and Mrs. Murray were being led down the hall by the nurse. Mrs. Murray was Dr. Wong's only patient for the day, being seen for a memory evaluation. Mr. Murray's posture was stooped, and he walked slowly, guiding his slightly disheveled wife into the exam room. Dr. Wong followed them in and shut the door. Within 15 minutes, I saw the red light outside the exam room come on, a signal that something is needed in the room. I told the nurses that I would check on Dr. Wong, as I thought she was likely trying to signal for me. When I opened the door, a wide-eyed Dr. Wong said, "I think he is having a stroke." I scanned Mrs. Murray sitting on the examination table, but nothing seemed amiss. "No, Dr. Kenny—*Mister* Murray."

Mr. Murray was slumped in the chair in the corner, his face slackened on the right side, his left arm loosely hanging, his words unintelligible. We called for the ambulance to take Mr. Murray to the emergency room and called the emergency contact (a neighbor) listed on the paperwork to care for Mrs. Murray. When the neighbor arrived, she told us that Mr. Murray had been doing his best to care for Mrs. Murray, but the strain was becoming too much. This appointment had been set up to begin to investigate options for both daytime and nighttime support. The Murrays had no other family. Sadly, Mr. Murray died from his stroke, and Mrs. Murray was emergently admitted to a long-term care facility.

The Murrays' situation illustrates the potential stress and its effect on physical health that may ensue from caregiving. Three-quarters of those who care for someone with dementia report concern for their health. There is a 41 percent increased risk of becoming frail from caring for a family member in their final year of dementia care. Evidence of how this may occur comes from studies showing an increase in physiologic biomarkers of chronic diseases that signify burden, such as higher stress hormones, high blood pressure, poor wound healing, and increased markers of cardiovascular risk. Similarly, those who care for someone with dementia are more likely to report their health as fair or poor compared with that of non-caregivers. This simple question of self-rated health is a strong predictor of future health care needs and mortality. In contrast, there are also studies showing that caregiving may be a positive experience, pointing to the hope that with a shift in focus away from the stressful aspects of caregiving, there is a way to offer love and support without self-harm.

## Caregiving Impact on Emotional Health

### RECOGNIZING THE POTENTIAL EMOTIONAL HEALTH CONSEQUENCES OF CAREGIVING
#### • *Sarah's Story* •

Sarah, a meek woman with stringy hair and wearing an oversized sweatshirt, approached the desk for our appointment. She was accompanied by her daughter, Jen, a taller, fashionable woman, who kept a loving hand on her mother's back. We sat in a quiet room, reviewing some of Sarah's mother's medical history before her recent transfer to the nursing home. Sarah's voice would catch off and on during parts of the story. I asked if Sarah was taking care of *herself* now that her mother's physical needs were being managed in the long-term care facility. Jen, who had not taken her hand off Sarah during the entire interview, sat up straighter and her eyes widened. Sarah said "yes" while Jen shook her head "no."

Jen prompted Sarah into saying that she spent all day at the assisted living facility, felt guilt and shame when she left, hadn't taken a vacation in eight years, had recent emergency surgery that did not resolve a stomach complaint, and was offered antianxiety medications by her primary care physician, who "didn't know what else to offer." As Sarah reported these facts about herself, her emotions ranged from flat, to angry, to tearful. Jen reported her own frustration that there was "no helping Mom understand that Grandma had needs, but so does she (Sarah)." We spent the next half hour talking about the benefits of therapy and an evaluation for depression. We discussed compassionate self-care so that Sarah would be able to continue to offer her mother excellent emotional care.

---

Caregiving (or care partnering) can be a wonderful emotional experience. Because of my mother's advanced disease, I learned to live from my heart in a new way. I learned to feel rather than think through a relationship. I learned to expand my ability to communicate non-verbally. And I learned to see love in someone's eyes in a new and marvelous way. But there was another side to that coin. I also needed to learn to feel and release grief—for the memories and loss of the personality who raised me, for the loss of hearing the stories of my childhood from someone who loved me more than anyone else. Finally, I needed to react to behaviors that were foreign to my relationship with my mother—her outbursts of anger, my impatience and fatigue.

Fifty-nine percent of family caregivers rate the emotional stress of caregiving as high or very high. This level of stress can lead to burnout and self-neglect. If the stress is not dealt with in healthy ways, caregivers are at increased risk of exhaustion, insomnia, and potentially depression. It is reported that 40 percent of caregivers suffer from depression, and the rates increase as the dementia and the family member's care needs increase. Depression has burdens of its own and can lead to alcohol or drug abuse, verbal or physical abuse of the family member, or neglect or premature transition to long-term care.

What can be done? Emotionally, the truth is a lot. But we must be willing to ask and receive. In her book *The Etiquette of Illness*, Susan P. Halpern relates a host of stories about communicating around illness. The stories are touching and enlightening, and, while they focus mostly on talking to people who have cancer, they can be useful for anyone dealing with a long-term chronic and disabling disease. They illustrate how to say "this is too much for me right now" so that you can ask for support from those around you in a positive way. They remind care partners to pause and become grounded before embarking into a care situation.

Suggestions for how to be able to do this include eating well, exercising, and being mindful. Nourishing your body with healthy foods and avoiding excess alcohol or drugs as a coping mechanism are excellent first practices in self-care. Exercise has been shown to be a tremendous stress reliever. Mountains of data on mindfulness practice, whether through meditation, prayer, or other methods, show that it brings about relaxation. Dr. Herbert Benson, a Harvard physician who pioneered research on meditation and the relaxation response, has shown that such practices result in less drug use, improvement in chronic diseases such as irritable bowel, reduced stress, less need for physician services, and better surgical outcomes.

## Caregiving and Relationships

### LOSING SHARED ACTIVITIES AND
### SHARED TIME TOGETHER
• *Dan and Shane's Story* •

Dan, a trim, compact man, sat in a wheelchair tightly gripping the armrests, his head bent so that his chin touched his chest. When approached, he would mutter obscenities punctuated by yelps telling others to get away from him. His son, Shane, a taller man than Dan but also trim and well-muscled, wanted to meet with me. Shane described his lifelong, close relationship with his father. He had admired his father's drive and ambition. They went into business together and owned multiple fitness centers. Working out together was a time to sweat and discuss the business. Dan's memory issues began as physical complaints, likely from Dan tensing his muscles to resist his anxieties about "losing it." He had tremendous headaches and backaches. Dan was now becoming easily irritated with Shane, something new and strange for Shane to deal with. Dan wasn't able to work out because of his memory and coordination issues. On many days, he was crippled by pain and could no longer even safely get to the business. Shane teared up as he described the loss of the father and the friendship that had been their day to day. He said he didn't know how to be with this "new man" who complained and snapped at him and could not seem to hold onto reason.

---

I doubt that a change in your relationship with your family member is a new concept to you in coming to terms with the end stages of Alzheimer disease and related dementia. As the dementia worsens, care required by family members or others increases. In addition, the shared experiences change. Some can keep a level of intimacy that was the same as before or potentially better, but most of the time, intimacy changes in a negative way. Sharing of memories, threads that previously connected the family, also changes. Along with the added burden of behavior disturbances that may accompany the disease, it is no wonder that most families experience stress and anxiety in their relationships. Nearly 20 percent of caregivers feel they have no choice but to deliver care, straining the relationship even further. The demands of caregiving increase as a person with dementia reaches the end of life, so that approximately 60 percent of caregivers feel they are under constant need to provide care.

## UNDERSTANDING DEMENTIA HELPS WITH COPING

What can be done to help? There is little research to help us answer this question, but studies suggest that combinations of understanding more about the disease process and how to work with the changes that accompany the disease provide a way forward. Education can assist in exploring new ways to continue your relationship with your family member. Questions may change from "Do you remember when . . . ?" to things that do not rely on memory such as "This picture reminds me of when we baked cookies together. Do you like the smell of cookies?"

I know that I learned to live more from my heart and in the moment with my mother in her late stages. I would comment on the slant of the sunlight or chill in the air during our walks outside, rather than bringing up plans for the future or asking her advice on how to manage the kids. I watched for her nonverbal cues to see if what I was talking about resonated with her. We spent more time looking closely at flowers or blades of grass, smelling and touching things together. We developed a new way to be close that didn't rely on words. I loved when we could connect through our eyes. She had to be well rested, and it wasn't always for long, but our forehead-to-forehead moments are now some of my most tender memories of my mother.

## SUPPORT GROUPS

Support groups can also be helpful. The relational connection that may be lost directly with your family member may be the commonality for making close and meaningful relationships with others. If you wonder what may be gained from a support group but are intimidated to join, try reading *The Caregivers* by Nell Lake. This book provides an intimate glance into caregiver support groups, how they work, and what relationships and advice may be gleaned from them. Several of my patients' family members report they were initially reluctant to join a support group, but it became a lifeline in coping with the journey of care partnering for dementia. The group can provide advice, support, experience, love—and occasionally tough love—when the challenges are out of balance with the pleasures of caregiving.

## ONLINE RESOURCES AND COMMUNITY

Online educational materials and support are also available. The Alzheimer's Association (www.alz.org), Health in Aging (www.healthinaging.org), and Family Caregiver Alliance (www.caregiver.org) are wonderful websites with a host of reliable information on dementia and in-home care for caregivers. Creating an online community is also possible. My sister related the story of a friend who used Facebook to ask for the things she needed for emotional (and other support) during her illness, her favorite request being funny cat videos! You can ask for anything you'd like from inspirational stories to tips on caregiving and activities that you think would be safe and supportive for you and your family member. Need a prayer—ask for it. A listening ear but no advice—ask for it. Women are often the caregivers, but women tend not to ask. Personal and societal reasons often keep women from asking too much, but once you know this, you can overcome it. In *Women Don't Ask*, Linda Babcock, a professor of economics at Carnegie Mellon University in Pittsburgh, Pennsylvania, outlines research on why women don't ask for what they need, want, and deserve at home or at work and then outlines strategies to begin to negotiate so that everyone's needs are met.

Online calendars and coordination centers allow others to know when you need meals or grocery shopping and offer updates in a secure way so that repeating the same message to concerned family and friends can be minimized. Examples of free and secure sites to consider are CaringBridge, a not-for-profit 501(c) organization that hosts personal, ad-free information (www.caringbridge.org), Lotsa Helping Hands (lostsahelpinghands.com), and Care Calendar (carecalendar.org).

The suggestion of creating an online support group may seem too overwhelming. Ask a friend or distant family member to take on this task and then train you. Or you can keep the support more low tech. Consider developing a simple phone tree. You call one or two people with requests or information, and they disseminate the request or information down the tree. Each person on the call tree contacts the next person on the list, and that person contacts the next person (and so on) until everyone on the call tree has been reached. If the next person on the list cannot be reached, the caller continues to the next level of the tree so that the chain does not break. To ensure that everyone who needs to know about the event has been notified, the last person on the call tree list should call the first person on the list to complete the loop. It is important that each person on the tree have up-to-date information and multiple phone numbers (cell, home, work) if needed.

## HONOR GIVING AND RECEIVING ASPECTS OF RELATIONSHIPS

Build your support system, and be creative in expanding it. Many individuals love to help but often don't know what is needed. There is much joy in giving. At times it is hard to learn to receive, but if you can understand that it brings purpose and meaning to others, you may be more likely to reach out. Joan Halifax, PhD, Buddhist teacher, Zen priest, anthropologist, and pioneer in the field of end-of-life care, performs an exercise in which two people walk together, one blindfolded while the other leads. Then the roles reverse. When leading, individuals report they feel strong, powerful, helpful, and open. When being led, individuals report feeling old, feeble, and overpowered. Hearing about this exercise helps me understand why individuals are reluctant to ask for help and guides me to find ways to equalize the giving/receiving relationship so that both parties benefit, including acknowledging that there may be initial feelings of loss of control. Understanding the dynamics in giving and receiving may open you to broadening your ability to request help and do so from a place of strength.

## IMPACT OF CAREGIVING ON WORK

The 2016 report from the Alzheimer's Association provides many statistics on caregivers. Often, caregivers change their work schedules to provide care in many ways, ranging from quitting their jobs (9%), taking a leave of absence (15%), reducing work to part time or taking a less demanding job (13%), taking an early retirement (8%), and turning down a promotion (7%). A majority (54%) report modifying time at work with coming in late, leaving early, or taking time off. Some (8%) report job performance suffering to the point of possible dismissal.

These sobering statistics easily demonstrate the potential for enormous financial repercussion. The estimated loss in wages, pension, and Social Security benefits are more than $300,000 over the caregiver's lifetime.

So what can be done to help?

### Federal Medical Leave Act

Protect your job security for needed time off by submitting a Federal Medical Leave Act form (www.dol.gov/whd/forms/WH-380-F.pdf) with your employer. You fill out a portion, and your family member's physician fills out the other parts. This can be a primary care physician or a specialist assisting with dementia diagnosis and care.

### Hire Help

Consider hiring someone to help with household responsibilities. Calculate your hourly pay, and if you can afford to hire someone to do something for you for less than that, this can be extremely helpful. Those responsible for care *can* do it all, but the responsibility is a burden. Can you hire someone to cook three meals per week for you and your family? The leftovers most likely will take you to a fourth night. Take out or food delivery may help with dinner another night. In my family, we had "breakfast for dinner" about twice a month and simple pasta with bottled marinara and salad twice a month, taking care of a sixth night without much difficulty. On Sundays, I would cook a meal with my mother in the kitchen with me. I usually made a roast or ham, something that I could turn into a soup or an easy tried-and-true meal like tacos or pulled pork in a barbecue sauce later in the week.

Assistance may be available for other household chores that don't require a personal touch, such as laundry. Is there a wash-and-fold service in your neighborhood? Or could you find someone to do this via Craigslist (www.craigslist.org)? If finances are tight and you don't mind doing laundry but hate cooking, maybe you could barter doing laundry for meal prep with a friend.

The next time you are talking about the weather or sports with work colleagues, ask them for their best kept secret for balancing work and family obligations. They may provide you with the "secret sauce" that clicks for you. I spent hours at the library when my children were young because of their age gap; one played in the children's area while I sat at a table helping another with homework and the third used the computer for educational games. During these times, I perused the shelves for books to help me cope with my work/family balance. One that struck me as both entertaining and spot on is *A Housekeeper Is Cheaper Than a Divorce* by Kathy Fitzgerald Sherman. She makes an excellent argument for choosing to hire someone to help with house management, so that time and energy away from work can be spent on relationships. The book outlines how to find, hire, and train a housekeeper. For someone managing work, caregiving, child-rearing, and personal sanity, it is a potential avenue not to be dismissed.

## Share Care with Others

Another movement that grew out of a friend's concern for a friend in need was Share the Care. The process of forming a community of helpers is outlined in a book by the same name by Cappy Capossela and Sheila Warnock. This guidebook could be used by a family to assist in caring for an individual with Alzheimer disease or dementia. It outlines how a community of caregivers can avoid the burnout that may accompany too few people involved in supporting someone whose care needs are complex. It wisely begins with exercises to bond the caregiving community and warns about potential resistance from primary caregivers who may not want to bring other caregivers into the mix for a host of reasons, including privacy and fear of losing their caregiving role. The book touches on dealing with the concerns and states firmly, as I believe, that if an individual or family can get beyond these concerns, a caregiving community will assist in ways beyond their wildest dreams. Small, daily decisions and burdens will be lifted.

A friend of mine, on receiving her diagnosis, relied on a few individuals, who until that time had been merely acquaintances. Her family situation was complex, as she was divorced, had teenage children, an elderly mother, and a brother with disabilities. Her illness and death, while on many levels full of growth for all of us involved, was also taxing because there were only a few of us, each with our own complex lives. If the community had been broadened and the responsibilities clearly delineated as outlined in Share the Care, I think we could have avoided some of the pain. I learned at least somewhat—but not enough—from this experience with my dear friend. At first, I still resisted help in my own journey with my mother, but I recognized that having her live in my home was not a good choice because of my other family and work responsibilities (three small children and being on-call for a hospital service). I did share responsibilities with my family—there was the legal expert, the financial expert, the connection/communication/relationship expert, a devoted soul that sent love and healing at all times, and me as the medical expert.

# TIPS FOR DAY-TO-DAY COPING, STRESS RELIEF, AND SELF-CARE

## Expanded View of the Disease

Remember that the journey of dementia can have many good moments mixed with the stresses. One gentleman with early stage Alzheimer disease organized and orchestrated an event that outlined his journey from diagnosis. He stated that he was initially angry but underwent a transformation to ultimately see his diagnosis as a gift—an opening to his creative side and a side that acknowledged the importance of relationships in his life. The event was very moving, with all of us in the room "seeing" the Alzheimer diagnosis from a different lens—an optimistic and open space for growth and discovery.

The gentleman's wife said that she had not progressed as far in her acceptance or view of the disease as had her husband. She admitted, with her husband as her guide, that she is beginning to see that the diagnosis has had some positive effects in their relationship and to change her view of the disease as more complex than the "terrible, depleting, soul-sucking" experience she envisioned on the day of the diagnosis. By more widely expanding her perspective, she was able to lift some of her original sense of burden. I admitted that I, too, guided by my mother and by patients in my practice, grew in a similar way. By seeing the disease as expansive in other aspects of life, I was open to all emotions and experiences and started finding that the good experiences often outweighed the bad. Labeling the experiences as "good or bad" dropped to a state of just "being" and acceptance—a much more positive way to go through my day to day.

## Moving Out of Isolation and into Society

Isolation may worsen the feelings of day-to-day stress. Movements for a dementia-friendly society are coming and are being implemented in the United States (www.dfamerica.org). The movement, which started in the United Kingdom, is an initiative dedicated to support families living with dementia by helping everyone in the community understand the complexities of dementia, by reducing fear, and by allowing access and inclusion for those living with dementia and their families. Research reveals that communities such as these enhance the well-being of individuals living with dementia and their care partners. Communities have safe and accessible transportation; businesses allow for appropriate, paced transactions; and entertainment includes abilities and interests of all, including those living with dementia.

---

### POINTS TO REMEMBER

▶ Family members provide the majority of care for an individual living with dementia. The care is unpaid and while it provides a sense of purpose, community and love, it also is accompanied by physical, emotional, financial, and relational strain.

▶ Although the physical health of a care partner may benefit from being active and engaged, poor health outcomes are more often reported from the physical and physiologic strains. Emotional strain may develop from caregiving, and it may increase as the dementia and care needs progress in your family member.

▶ Your relationship with your family member living with dementia will be constantly changing. You may need to develop other relationships to support you during this phase in the journey with dementia.

▶ Learning more about dementia, its typical progression, and caregiving tips may ease some of the stress from the unpredictability of care and the chronicity of the responsibilities. Several reputable websites and resources are available and outlined in the chapter.

---

### ACTION PLAN

▶ Learn what you can about dementia and the progression of the disease to assist you in planning and preparing upcoming care needs.

▶ Combat the statistics of the burden of caregiving on the physical and emotional health by good self-care, including nutrition, healthy behaviors such as exercise and only moderate alcohol consumption. Caregivers should not neglect their own health, in terms of both preventive practices and attention to current health problems.

▶ Practice stress-reducing activities such as meditation or engage in an activity that allows personal relaxation (such as painting or singing).

▶ Watch for signs of depression, such as insomnia, irritability, exhaustion, lack of enjoyment in any activity, crying, or turning to alcohol or drugs to cope. If these signs appear, contact your physician for assistance and possibly referral.

▶ Consider a support group or building a care community and explore ways to assist your needs balancing care and working outside the home.

──────────  ADDITIONAL READING AND RESOURCES  ──────────

▶ *The Caregivers: A Support Group's Stories of Slow Loss, Courage, and Love*, by Nell Lake

This book of stories from a support group focuses on caregivers' personal challenges, providing support to common caregiver stories and themes. It also provides a glimpse into a caregiver support group so that one may decide if the process may be right for them.

▶ *Share the Care: How to Organize a Group to Care for Someone Who Is Seriously Ill*, by Cappy Capossela and Sheila Warnock

This guidebook discusses how to build a community, or group, to help support a family caring for someone with a long-term, intensive illness. The book provides exercises to assist the group in finding an identity and in respecting the needs of each other and those being supported.

# Active Dying

How can families recognize the transition to active dying? This chapter describes the signs and symptoms that are common in the final days to weeks of life and how these may change in the final hours. It will help you understand the typical treatments that are offered in the final days. Numerous examples will show you how friends and families experience, cope with, and celebrate these final days.

## RECOGNIZING THE START OF ACTIVE DYING
### • *The Kenny Family Story* •

"She's in the beauty parlor." I was a bit surprised. I was visiting my mom three times a day lately, partly to ensure that her wish not to eat was honored by any new caregiver who might not know or agree with her wishes, but mostly because I knew her days in this world were limited. The day before, her head flopped to the left and right, although her eyes followed me perfectly. The inability to hold her head upright meant she would likely be with us for only hours to days rather than days to weeks. She sat in the beauty parlor, head flopped to the side with beautifully coiffed hair but panting and struggling to catch her breath. I quickly wheeled her back to her room and lifted her into her bed.

Her hospice nurse had heard of Mom's recent changes and was on the spot. She immediately recognized signs of active dying— quick, short breaths associated with a rattling noise, moans, and restlessness. She turned to me, grasped that I also knew the end was near—and then we both began to laugh at the absurdity of the dying woman in the beauty parlor. Giggling, we acknowledged that her hair looked great. It was my mother's way. She needed to leave us looking good. And she would. We raised the head of the bed to help my mother breathe and to stabilize her floppy neck. The nurse began administering morphine for my mom's shortness of breath and fidgeting, a sign of the discomfort she was feeling. I called my brothers and sister; no one was shocked by the call after recent visits confirming weight loss, sleepiness, and Mom's overall decline. Mom's neighbor's family members sat with me at her bedside to offer support and to thank us for allowing them to share the experience and guidance as they prepared to face a similar situation.

---

I have been fortunate to be led to work I love and am suited for. In medical school, a series of lectures during my second year on geriatric medicine "spoke" to me, and I knew it was my path. During a hospice rotation, I was given an audiotaped lecture on signs and symptoms at the time of death, delivered by two hospice nurses. My instructor warned me that some of the information on the audio was "a bit out there" but that the information on recognizing active dying was sound and solid, and he asked that I keep an open mind. I loved what I heard on that audiotape, and I remember that it confirmed what I had experienced in my life—that dying was usually a peaceful process and could be used as a time to experience wonder, growth, and joy along with sadness and grief.

The book *Final Gifts*, by Maggie Callanan and Patricia Kelley, outlines the "out there" information I heard on the audiotape: that individuals who are dying talk symbolically about moving on, that they often see or sense guides to assist in transitioning from this life, and that death is peaceful and accepted by most. I have found that sharing my stories of experiences around death of others, as Callanan and Kelley do in their book, with my patients and their families, provides comfort and helps individuals and families cope with and accept dying.

The death of my father highlights some of these messages. During my sophomore year of high school, I had a premonition of his death. In the next few months, my quiet and nondemonstrative father reached out to create memories and one-on-one experiences with many of his children. He joined a bowling league with my sister and attended Weight Watchers meetings with me, both activities uncharacteristic for him. He organized a wonderful 30th wedding anniversary party for my mother. The celebration was at our house, and friends and family from across the country attended. The next morning, when my father never woke, my mother was surrounded by loving support to assist her with his death.

The story of my father's death is typical of other stories I've heard. Although my father had not been ill and died unexpectedly in his sleep, there were changes that suggested, on some level, he knew he was going to die and worked to put some relationships in order. Some of this ordering of events may be lost when one is in the end stages of dementia, but it is not uncommon to hear that restlessness subsides after a visit from an estranged family member or after a milestone such as a graduation or birth of a grandchild.

---

## MAKING TREATMENT DECISIONS AT THE END
### • *Karen and Toby's Story* •

Karen, friendly but reserved, asked to meet with me to assist in decision making about her father, Toby. The focus in the house had been Trisha, Karen's mother, who had battled mental health issues, complicating her life, and then her care and death from a rapidly aggressive cancer. Toby had been the peacekeeper in the family, tending to Trisha's needs and demands for years. Once she was gone, Karen realized Toby's cognitive abilities were markedly impaired. Since his wife's death, it became apparent that Toby could not live alone and needed assistance with most of his activities of daily living. He was rapidly losing weight and was beginning to fall often. Karen was feeling guilty that she had missed signs of her father's decline and needs. After reassuring Karen that the structure that Trisha insisted on may have helped Toby function day to day, Karen began asking several questions about making decisions for Toby so that she would be better prepared for his life course and not be caught off guard, as she had been for her mother's death.

Karen was put off by the aggressive treatment given to her mother, the stay in the intensive care unit, and the never-ending complications and resuscitation needed over the last few weeks of her mother's life. "I can't imagine putting my father through something similar. It just seems wrong." Karen asked pointed, informed questions about reversible causes of dementia, whether (and how much) of Toby's decline could be due to grief or depression, treatment options, and the typical course for decline. Near the end of the visit, Karen hesitated and fidgeted, and I asked if there was anything else. "I don't know how to ask." There was a long pause. "Is it always like with my mom?" "Are you asking if dying is always like it happened for your mother?" I asked. Karen looked embarrassed, eyes downcast, voice low as she answered meekly, "Yes."

---

Talking of death can seem scary or taboo. Most people have not witnessed a death, often being whisked out of the room if it occurs in a hospital setting or sheltered from it by family. Many are afraid of what they will see. Death has not often occurred in the home in the past century, tending more to happen in some type of health care setting. However, with the emergence of the hospice movement in the mid-nineteenth century, death is beginning to occur more often at home, at least in those diagnosed with cancer. But this is not the trend for those with dementia. Two-thirds of individuals who die with dementia do so in a nursing home.

One common question I am asked by family members is, "What will the death be like at the end?" The weeks before death from dementia are often accompanied by a further change in function with more weakness, dependence, fatigue and sleep, less interest in food or drink, more withdrawal in eye contact and concentration. This description is much like the preceding months in the later stages of dementia.

In the final days to hours (active dying), the individual will have periods of unresponsiveness, glassy eyes and unfocused pupils, abnormal respiratory patterns, low blood pressure, cold extremities, and mottling of skin. There may be sounds of congested breathing. The individual may seem to have a period of increased energy seen as agitation or lucidity, at times with speech even if he or she has not spoken in a long time. The cause for this is unknown, but it is reported by many hospice personnel and families. Table 9.1 lists common characteristics of active dying and how to approach it.

**TABLE 9.1** Common Characteristics of Active Dying

| TIMING | SYMPTOM | APPROACH |
| --- | --- | --- |
| Weeks prior | Increased sleep and withdrawal | Allow for sleep and be sensitive to need for quiet |
| | Loss of interest in foods and fluids | Offer food and liquids for pleasure |
| | | Be attentive to mouth care; offer moisture to lips and mouth |
| | Restlessness | Be attentive for signs or causes and respond |
| | | Consider pain, fatigue, and spiritual/relational angst; offer comforting words and permission to die |
| Days prior | Decreased response to external stimuli, glassy eyed, unfocused | No action required |

**TABLE 9.1** (*continued*)

| TIMING | SYMPTOM | APPROACH |
|---|---|---|
| Days prior (*continued*) | Changes in breathing, including terminal congestion or death rattle | Oxygen if provides comfort |
| | | Fan to provide breeze across face |
| | | Medication, such as morphine, if breathing labored |
| | | Drying agent (hyoscyamine, glycopyrrolate, scopolamine, or atropine) will assist with sounds in terminal congestion, but this is of more benefit for those at the bedside than the individual with terminal congestion |
| | Low blood pressure with cold, mottled extremities | No action required |
| | Potential surge of energy | Safe, supportive environment |

## RECOGNIZING THE "TYPICAL" DYING PROCESS

### • *The Winston Family Story* •

Mr. and Mrs. Winston both lived with dementia—Mr. Winston with vascular dementia and Mrs. Winston with probable Alzheimer dementia. They had four funny, loving, smart, and smart-alecky devoted daughters who lifted the mood and energy of any room. These women were phenomenal at "natural care partnering." They allowed their parents independence as long as possible and took turns being the "heavy" when new services or support needed to be added despite their parents' resistance. Mr. Winston died quickly and quietly in his sleep. The daughters, while sad, were grateful for their father's peaceful passing. Soon after, their mother began a more rapid decline, and they knew she was nearing the end of her life as well. They each applied for the Federal Medical Leave Act at their jobs so they could share in their mother's final care at home.

The first few months, they fell into a nice rhythm of working in a tag-team manner, sitting with their mother, caring for one another's children, and making meals to be split between households while their mother napped. There were bumps in the road. Mrs. Winston would become restless in the late afternoon and yell out or resist care. The daughters watched for clues to what was causing the problems. They tried soothing music, encouraging a nap earlier in the day, and several other strategies. A scowl was more and more often on Mrs. Winston's face, which was unusual for her and did not abate despite a trial of pain medications. An antidepressant in low dose did lessen the restlessness, yelling, and scowl within a few weeks. The daughters suspected Mrs. Winston missed her husband. She became weaker and weaker and would not eat even small bites when offered. The daughters described her as "disconnected" much of the time. Then, as if she was suddenly infused with Herculean strength, Mrs. Winston began getting out of bed and walked halfway across the room and started mumbling. The daughters were able to make out the word "key" in her speech. They recognized that the spurt of power might be a signal of the end and thought perhaps the reference to a key represented a need to find her way to death. They took turns talking to their mother over the next day or so. "We love you, Mom." "Dad has the key and will help you." "You've done such a wonderful job raising me and blessing me with my sisters—you've done everything for us."

As Mrs. Winston slipped into a quiet unconsciousness, the daughters sat and talked together, laughing about how their parents "in heaven" would do such a good job keeping an eye on them in new ways. They discussed the favorite stories about their parents they planned to tell on birthdays and holidays to keep Grammy and Gramps alive in their children's eyes. Mrs. Winston's breathing became very irregular. It started deep and labored and then stopped for seconds at a time. When it started again, it was soft and slow and then built back up to deep and labored. The daughters whispered their goodbyes and sang the chorus to "Good Night, Irene" together, a song their mother loved. They stayed together laughing, crying, hugging, and reminiscing until Mrs. Winston took her final breath.

---

The Winstons' story illustrates several common occurrences of someone's final days: lethargy and weakness, unresponsiveness, restlessness, a burst of energy, and irregular and congested breathing. The daughters were well versed in self-care and support and had seen someone die before, so their anxiety or fear around the process was lessened. They were able to make the experience special in their own family's way by discussing traditions for their children in their mother's presence so that Mrs. Winston could hear them, singing a playful but meaningful song to "send their mother off," and expressing a full range of emotions in the room. During the time of restlessness in the day before Mrs. Winston's death, the family sought for meaning and insight in her actions and words that may have given her permission to go and assurance that all would be well for them. They also looked for the best way to comfort her restlessness, not resorting immediately to sedating medications, in the months before her death, finally concluding that it was unresolved grief (although they had explored the possibility of pain and uncomfortable situations such as fatigue or hunger). This type of intentional approach and exploration is often rewarded with a smoother transition to death.

---

## DEALING WITH FRIGHTENING SYMPTOMS
## AND LETTING HOSPICE HELP

### • *Mrs. Gordon and Susan's Story* •

Mrs. Gordon's daughter Susan called me in a panic. "You have to come over. Mom is seeing her husband. He's been gone over 20 years! She is frightened. I am frightened." Susan was the only caregiver to Mrs. Gordon, a feisty, in-charge woman, all of ninety pounds soaking wet. Mrs. Gordon had been deteriorating over the last year. She had lost more and more function and was not stable walking. She had lost her appetite and always seemed to be losing two pounds, but then pushing milkshakes to gain back one. She kept her voice during her decline. Although she wasn't always oriented, her vascular dementia had spared her ability to make her wishes known. When I visited, she reported seeing her late husband but refused to let him in. "He wants me to go with him, but what would happen to Susan?" Mrs. Gordon did not like her husband there and asked repeatedly to send him away; she was not aware that he was a hallucination. Mrs. Gordon, Susan, and I discussed hospice care, but Mrs. Gordon would not allow Susan to let anyone in the house to help.

The visions of her husband and occasionally her parents went on for a few months as Mrs. Gordon alternately lost weight and struggled to drink milkshakes "like medicine" to make up the pounds. Susan was strained by the caregiving and stress of the visions, the weight loss, the functional loss, and the inevitability that Mrs. Gordon's time was limited. Mrs. Gordon's word was final in Susan's eyes, so if her mother said she would fight to live, they both took up the charge. I spoke to each of them alone and together about letting go. At one point, Mrs. Gordon allowed hospice to start but discharged the nurses within a day. Mrs. Gordon stated, "I'm not ready for that!" Over and over, Mrs. Gordon and Susan agreed that it was time to switch to a comfort approach, but then I would receive a call the next day imploring we try one more thing, one more trick to buy more time. This struggle went on for months. Mrs. Gordon fell and was in pain often, but any attempt to treat her pain made her cognition worse, and she resisted. Her primary wishes were to be as clear as possible and alive for Susan. Then, one fateful day, she had a severe fall and injured her back. She developed delirium while in the emergency room and returned home agitated and in extreme pain. Despite wanting to continue the fight to live, Mrs. Gordon had run out of energy. Her breathing became more labored, and her extremities cold and blue. Susan's fear of the changes she saw in her mother grew, and she allowed hospice to be called.

The hospice team assisted Mrs. Gordon with her pain and labored breathing, successfully keeping her comfortable in her final days. The nurses explained the changes, including the mottling skin and irregular breathing, and comforted Susan as her mother died. The nursing staff coached Susan so that she understood that morphine helped with pain and breathlessness and was not "stopping Mom's breathing or causing her death." Other medications were used to dry the congestion that causes a "death rattle" in the final day of Mrs. Gordon's life. And the hospice team provided bereavement counseling for Susan for the next 13 months as she relived each decision she and her mother had made in Mrs. Gordon's struggle to remain alive as long as possible.

---

This story, too, exemplifies common occurrences during the months before death. Mrs. Gordon found the presence of her husband disturbing, keeping him outside, cold and unhappy while he waited for her. She seemed to have unresolved issues about meeting him, because she did not want to leave her daughter. Susan was also conflicted, wanting to spare her mother suffering but not wanting to lose her. The conflict was borne out in initially calling in hospice but then immediately reversing that decision. Thankfully, the hospice team returned to assist Mrs. Gordon in her final week and to support and comfort Susan about signs associated with death.

Further information on hospice can be found in chapter 6, "Decisions about Places of Care." Hospice teams consist of physician, nurses, social workers, health care aids, chaplains, spiritual counselors, volunteers, and other support individuals who all share a common concern and expertise in assisting in the dying process. The focus of the team is on comfort and peace for the dying individual and his or her family. The team's expertise in difficult conversations and experience in handling the physical, emotional, and spiritual ups and downs common at the end of life are key for many families weathering a challenging time in their lives.

---

### FORESHADOWING DEATH

#### • *Joy's Story* •

Joy sat in the same chair in the dining room every day. She could not remember much of her daily events or the people who partnered in her care, but she loved how she looked, focusing on the sparkle in her outfits, the rouge on her cheeks, and the perfect color on her nails. Although she rarely spoke, she smiled often, particularly at an outfit she liked on a visitor. Unflattering outfits received a frown, providing the clue I needed to purge a few pieces of clothing from my closet.

After a Sunday outing, I tucked my mother into bed as she was exhausted and developing a cold. As I waited to report the cold symptoms to the nurse, I found Joy sitting in the common room. Joy told me that her husband (who had been dead for 10 years) was coming back in a moment to sit with her. "He's getting ready for our trip. I'm so excited." I assumed Joy meant her son, who wasn't able to visit often because of his work schedule. Joy continued, "He loves me so much and says we will be going in the next few days." I told Joy everyone loved her and that her smile was a bright light. I had never heard Joy speak so clearly or so much. When the nurse was available, I mentioned how talkative Joy had been. The nurse was surprised as she hadn't heard it and reported that Joy's son had not been there. The next day, Joy spoke to two others, once again reporting that her husband was planning a trip for her. On the third day, Joy could not be aroused from sleep. Her son came to sit with her, and she died peacefully a few hours later.

---

Joy's story exemplifies the symbolic changes that may foreshadow death. She usually did not speak but then talked about her husband coming to travel with her. Not all people believe that this can happen, but it is well described in *Final Gifts* by Maggie Callanan and Patricia Kelley. I have also seen it many times. Listening symbolically is often helpful in understanding the needs of those who have lost their voice to dementia. I had a patient who spoke, over and over, of being pregnant. Her family felt she was delusional and requested medication. I wondered what would make her think she was pregnant. Potentially persistent nausea? I stopped a common medication for dementia that causes nausea—and her pregnancy vanished!

My mother, a usually happy and playful soul, began to frown and scowl at everything. She rolled her eyes at her neighbors when they spoke, she stopped joining in during sing-a-longs, she pushed food around on her plate, and she started refusing toileting and bathing assistance. The staff wondered if she needed an antipsychotic so that she would allow help with personal care. But I looked at the bigger picture. My mother had stopped participating in activities that she usually enjoyed—singing, socializing, and eating. She looked angry when she usually wore a smile. We tried an antidepressant, and the results were excellent. My mother's smile returned, and she became the easygoing, cooperative, impish woman that she'd always been. The message here is that you know your family member better than anyone. Helping to discover the potential meanings behind puzzling words or actions may make the difference in choosing an approach or medication to maximize comfort.

## COMMON SYMPTOMS DURING ACTIVE DYING AND HELPFUL APPROACHES/MEDICATIONS

*Pain* and its assessment may change as the end of life approaches, but pain should still be treated aggressively. Behavioral signs may indicate the presence of pain. These behaviors may include frowning, clenching of the jaw, drawing up the legs, rigid or jerking movements, crying, and moaning or whimpering. Attempts to console the individual may be less effective than they were previously.

Narcotic pain medications are often given during the final stages of dying. They can be given by mouth, rectally, through a skin patch, or by injection under the skin or intravenously. Possible side effects include delirium and a jerking or twitching of the arms or legs. Changing to a different narcotic can relieve these symptoms (if death is not imminent). Narcotics can alter consciousness, but impending death usually does as well. Family members should consult with the health care staff to help differentiate between these two situations. If the medication is decreased or held to try to make this determination, everyone should stay alert for behavioral evidence of pain so that comfort is ensured.

*Shortness of breath* occurs in 70 percent of dying individuals. It is usually caused by several factors, so varied approaches may be needed to address it. Someone being present can be helpful, as can a soothing voice, gentle touch, relaxation techniques, a breeze over the face (created with a fan), an open window, or supplemental oxygen. Medications that may be helpful include those for anxiety and opioid analgesics (such as morphine). Sometimes, morphine is withheld because of fear that it can cause respiratory depression, especially in those who have a history of lung disease. However, morphine is such an effective and helpful treatment for shortness of breath, it can be used effectively by adjusting the dose to achieve a rate of 12–20 breaths per minute. Most shortness of breath can be managed with these few interventions.

More breathing changes may occur as death is nearing. A pattern of abnormal breathing may be seen, with cycles of increasingly deeper breaths and then shallow breaths, followed by a pause in breathing (called apnea). There may be a snort or gasp when the cycle begins again.

*Terminal congestion,* which is also called the "death rattle," is caused by moisture in the airway combined with weakness of the airway muscles so that the moisture is not cleared away. It usually does not bother the individual who is dying but is often troubling or distressing to family members. If the person is positioned on his or her side, gravity can help clear the secretions. If this doesn't help, medication can be given to dry the secretions.

*Dry mouth* is the only symptom of dehydration bothersome to someone who is dying. The other aspects of dehydration, including decreased secretions and urination, less nausea and vomiting, and less risk of heart failure, ascites, and edema, are welcome to ease the transition to death. The mouth and lips are cared for by swabbing the mouth with water or glycerin, lubricating the mouth with sips or sprays of water or saliva substitutes, and lubricating the lips with moisturizer or petroleum jelly. Commercial mouth moisturizers may last a little longer. A room humidifier may also be helpful.

*Cold extremities and skin mottling* are seen as death nears because the blood supply centers on the body's major organs (heart, lungs, liver), leaving the arms and legs cool and the skin discolored in lace-like patches. It is not painful, and usual skin care is indicated.

*Terminal agitation or delirium* occurs in about 10 percent of dying individuals within the last few hours of life and can vary in presentation from disorientation to restlessness to more pronounced agitation with yelling and flailing. It is important to look for conditions that may cause discomfort, such as pain or distended bladder. If none is found, anxiety is common as death nears and may be approached by ensuring a calm and supportive environment. If further support is required, medications that help with anxiety may be used.

---

## STAYING CLOSE IN THE FINAL STAGES
### • *The Raymonds' Story* •

I sat at my mother's bedside, reading aloud. She was deep in sleep or in a light coma. She was in her final days. A tap on the door and the question, "May I join you?" came from my friend Becky. We had become friends when our children were in preschool, two working professionals balancing child-rearing and professional advancement. In summer, we would take the kids from preschool to her parents' house to swim in their pool. We all loved having deep conversations sitting at poolside, doling out popsicles and dodging the occasional splash of a cannonball.

The Raymonds now lived in the same assisted living community as my mother. Mrs. Raymond had dementia due to Parkinson disease, and Mr. Raymond had probable mixed dementia complicated by depression. Becky was kind and big hearted, but as the decision maker for both, she was also direct, inquisitive, and systematic in data collection and decisive. She came to my mother's bedside to offer me comfort but also to gather information on how to be with someone who is dying. She stopped in often during the last two months of my mother's life. Becky saw me sitting quietly, holding my mother's hand, reading to her from different books, singing with her while she hummed or just raised an eyebrow. She saw me sitting and meditating next to my mother. What Becky couldn't see was that I was breathing in the pain of the loss and breathing out loving kindness—for my mother, for myself, for all who live with dementia, for their families.

"Mom likes it quiet now as she seems to be half with us and half in another place, away from here. She gets annoyed at times when I pull her back here to me," I told Becky. Becky said she was noticing the same thing with her mom. After my mother died, I visited Becky in her parents' apartment. "Thank you for sharing your family's journey with us. I've learned to slow down and be quieter with my parents. It seems strange, but there is a feeling of closeness now. We focus on each other, rather than on the next thing that needs to be done. Even though they speak so little, I feel we are closer."

---

## SUGGESTIONS FOR HOW TO SIT AT THE BEDSIDE

The Raymonds' story illustrates what I see time and again. People are often not comfortable sitting at the bedside. They don't know what to say or what to do. Sitting quietly does not occur commonly in our society. We brag about how busy we are or how we don't have time to [fill in the blank]. Our busyness is often seen as a badge of honor.

Shelf after shelf of self-help books direct us to spend our time efficiently and productively.

Slowing down to sit at the bedside can serve many purposes though. It allows time to reflect on the upcoming passing of the person before you. It allows time to say the things you may want to express, in words, whispers, thoughts, or writing. Ira Byock, MD, author and director of Palliative Care at Dartmouth Hitchcock Medical Center, states in his book *The Four Things That Matter Most* that there is emotional healing power in conveying certain truths to those we love or care for: "Please forgive me," "I forgive you," "Thank you," and "I love you." He posits those we care for don't always know the obvious and that stating it explicitly leads to healing, growth, or completion. Byock concedes that the four phrases will not magically make relationships heal or expand (although they may) but suggests that the simplicity and the directness of the four phrases opens the door either for communication or compassion. I believe that the intention is conveyed to those with dementia, even when we are unsure whether the meaning of the words is missed. When an individual is in a coma and cannot speak or respond physically, there is evidence that they remain able to hear.

This may be a time to just sit and read aloud, perhaps beautiful poetry or from a book you love. Maybe something funny, such as a book of jokes, or something touching, such as the *Chicken Soup for the Soul*–type of writings. My mother loved sentimental, touching, or tender writings. These types of stories reached into her and evoked emotion, shown by a tear running down her face. I knew that she had made a connection, providing me with hope that, at other times, I, too, was making a heart-to-heart connection with her.

Just sitting may be what is required. Joan Halifax, PhD, author, and Buddhist monk, specializing in contemplative care at the end-of-life, writes in her book *Being with Dying* that many of us feel that "silence and stillness aren't good enough when suffering is present." She states that we feel we must do something or move in some way— clean, talk, pace, work. She suggests that just sitting there can open a tender connection. Listening and being present are big gifts. Those with advanced dementia may not speak much, but when they do—with their eyes or their words—will we be quiet enough to hear them? And then, can we react by simply observing our reaction and letting it pass while we stay present for the individual dying?

## DEATH AT HOME

Nothing has to be done immediately after a person's death. Take the time you need. Some people want to stay in the room with the deceased; others prefer to leave. You might want to have someone make sure the body is lying flat before the joints become stiff and cannot be moved. This rigor mortis begins sometime during the first hours after death.

After the death, how long you can stay with the deceased may depend on where death happens. If it happens at home, there is no need to move the body right away. This is the time for any special religious, ethnic, or cultural customs that are performed soon after death.

If the death seems likely to happen in a facility, such as a hospital or a nursing home, discuss any important customs or rituals with the staff early on, if possible. That will allow them to plan so you can have the appropriate time with the body.

Some families want time to sit quietly with the deceased, console one another, and share memories. You could ask a member of your religious community or a spiritual counselor to come. If you have a list of people to notify, this is the time to call those who might want to come and see the body before it is moved.

Soon after, the death must be officially pronounced by a qualified individual, such as a doctor or a hospice nurse. This person also fills out the forms certifying the cause, time, and place of death. These steps will make it possible for an official death certificate to be prepared. This legal form is necessary for many reasons, including life insurance and financial and property issues.

If hospice is helping, a plan for what happens after death should already be in place. If death happens at home without hospice, try to talk with the doctor, local medical examiner (coroner), your local health department, or a funeral home representative in advance about how to proceed.

Arrangements should be made to pick up the body as soon as the family is ready and according to local laws. Usually this is done by a funeral home. The hospital or nursing facility, if that is where the death took place, may call the funeral home for you. If at home, you will need to contact the funeral home directly or ask a friend or family member to do that for you.

The doctor may ask if you want an autopsy. This is a medical procedure conducted by a specially trained physician to learn more about what caused the death. For example, if the person who died was believed to have Alzheimer disease, the examination of brain tissue collected during the autopsy will allow for a definitive diagnosis. If your religion or culture objects to autopsies, talk to the doctor. Some people planning a funeral with a viewing worry about having an autopsy, but the physical signs of an autopsy are usually hidden by clothing.

When there is a medical emergency, such as a heart attack, stroke, or serious accident, we know to call 911. But if a person is dying at home and does not want CPR (cardiopulmonary resuscitation), calling 911 is not necessary. In fact, a call to 911 could cause confusion. In many areas, the EMTs (emergency medical technicians) who respond to 911 calls are required to perform CPR if someone's heart has stopped. Consider having a non-hospital do-not-resuscitate (DNR) order if the person is dying at home, indicated by a bracelet, so that if someone does call 911, an unwanted resuscitation attempt is not made.

## RIGHT TO DIE OR ASSISTED DEATH

The movement to allow individuals to choose their right to die rests on the premise that every competent adult has the right to humankind's ultimate civil and personal liberty—the right to die in a manner and at a time of their own choosing. From this right, the best, safe, and effective methods of death require the assistance of a physician via access to medications. Hence, the emergence of the term *assisted death*, or *assisted suicide*. After a patient-initiated request, a physician provides the means for the individual to end her or his own life. This is legal in only a few states. Oregon was the first to pass the Death with Dignity Act in 1994. Other states currently with legislation allowing physician-assisted death include Washington, Vermont, Colorado, Washington, DC, Montana, and California. Each state has guidelines, but all mandate that the individual be terminally ill and competent. These laws do not pertain to an individual with dementia, because their competence or capacity would be questioned.

Euthanasia is the painless killing of a person suffering from an incurable and painful disease. This practice is illegal in the United States.

---

## POINTS TO REMEMBER

▸ Dying is usually a peaceful process. With information, patience, tools, and support, the process can also be a time, along with the sorrow, of transformation, growth, and even joy for families.

▸ Individuals may signal their time of death is approaching with visions of deceased family members or places and symbolic language of travel or transformation.

▸ Discussing the usual course of death aids many individuals or family members in making informed choices on how to handle the typical process of death in a calm and informed way.

▸ Typical symptoms in the weeks before death include weakness, increased sleep, limited attention span, loss of interest in food or drink, difficulty swallowing, increased disorientation.

▸ The symptoms of impending death (in the few days to hours preceding) include altered consciousness, glassy eyes, abnormal respiration, cool extremities, low blood pressure and pulse, terminal congestion, and terminal agitation.

▶ Several common sense strategies and a few medications may decrease symptoms at end of life.

▶ As a family member, finding the courage to sit at the bedside can open an intimate connection with the individual who is dying. Time at the bedside can be spent in whatever way is meaningful for all involved.

---

### ACTION PLAN

▶ If you have had limited exposure to people dying, consider reading a book such as *Final Gifts* (see "Additional Reading and Resources") to help prepare you for when the time comes.

▶ During a family get-together, discuss your intentions for the final hours for your family. Do you want any special messages or send-offs, poems, songs, religious ceremonies? Plan them now, gather whatever materials will be needed, and keep them accessible (e.g., a nearby closet).

---

### ADDITIONAL READING AND RESOURCES

▶ *Final Gifts*, by Maggie Callanan and Patricia Kelley

This book, filled with stories from the experiences of two hospice nurses, is about the messages and legacies left by those who are dying. It helps readers expand their awareness of the experience that occurs at the end of life and gives examples of responses.

▶ *The Four Things That Matter Most*, by Ira Byock

Dr. Byock, a palliative care physician, describes how using four simple phrases (*Please forgive me, I forgive you, Thank you, and I love you*) have aided in relationships of people and their families who are coping with dying and the end of life. He gives examples of how the words can lead to healing, forgiveness, and reconnection.

# Afterloss and Adjustment

When a family member dies, the caregiver undergoes a transition. From the early days of grief, caregivers need to move through acute grief and learn to recognize when their grief may have veered in an unhealthy direction. Although caregivers lose their caregiving role, it is a time to recognize and celebrate the tremendous growth that accompanies some of the heartache that travels along with caregiving.

---

### GRIEVING AND THE LOSS OF CAREGIVING
#### • The Kenny Family Story •

I sat on the couch. Constantly. It was as if I had sprouted roots that grew through the springs, through the floor, and into the ground. My kids would climb up next to me, hug me, push a cup of tea into my hand. I stared out the window, watched the snow fall, listened to the silence of winter, cried, and asked my family to take messages since I wouldn't answer the phone or the door. I vacillated between exhaustion, sadness, and boredom with my exhaustion and sadness. This was grief for me. As I began to talk more, I told my oldest son I was thinking about adopting a child. He, thankfully, leaned in close and whispered, "Just wait, Mom. I think you just miss Grandma so much you want to fill the hole."

How could I not have seen it? There was a hole, both in my heart for my mom and in my time for the caregiving that I had come to identify with. The busy was gone. The juggling had ended. My kids had grown up and definitely become independent while I had been spending more time with my mother. Now was the time to honor the grief for the love of my mom—a process that would take time and tenderness. It was time to let go of the caregiving.

It would take courage to not fill the hole with more caregiving but instead to explore a new way. The final gift my mother gave me was the gift of receiving. She had modeled how to be taken care of as she left this world, slowly and gracefully. I had incorporated the lesson, adding it to my tool box for a fuller and richer life. I grew as a mother, a friend, and a lover because I learned to receive.

## RESILIENCE IN GRIEF

New research in understanding bereavement has started to focus on caregivers, because most deaths (70%) occur in individuals that had one or more chronic conditions that required care. The research reveals that caregivers show resilience in adapting to the death of a family member. Most individuals have a period of sadness and more depressive symptoms, but these decrease within a month of the death and return to near normal levels within a year of the death. Theories for the rapid recovery include time to do some of the work of grieving before the death (anticipatory grief), fatigue from, and therefore relief from caregiving (which allows for some release of guilt because "I've done what I could") and finally, time and realization that the death is coming.

Developing resilience at the time of a death can be done in a host of ways. Strategies to assist with getting through the acute grief include finding laughter and joy amid the sadness, selecting and focusing on fond memories, seeking and finding the silver lining, and taking time to reflect on and appreciate life. Although most adults are resilient, those who had been involved with caring for an individual with dementia are less likely to recover as well. In this group, 20 to 30 percent have a prolonged, complicated grief, while those whose family member died of an illness other than dementia have only a 10 percent rate of complicated grief.

# ANTICIPATORY GRIEF

---

## ADJUSTING TO CHANGES, KNOWING MORE IS TO COME
### • *The Mayfields' Story* •

Bob, the oldest son of Dr. Bob, called me the Monday morning after Thanksgiving. "Dr. Kenny, may I speak to you about Mom?" I was surprised. I cared for his father, a wonderful, kind, scholarly physician who was living with dementia. His wife, Amanda, was his biggest supporter and advocate. She remained one step behind Dr. Bob with an uncanny ability to foster independence but be unobtrusively there for support if needed.

Bob said, "At Thanksgiving, Mom pulled off her usual beautiful dinner, but she's thin and quiet, and I caught her in the kitchen weeping. She insists nothing is wrong, but when I pushed her she said she's worried about Dad. What should we do? We're worried about her, and she won't leave Dad to go to the doctor." Bob said he could bring his parents in that day. Amanda usually brought notes about Dr. Bob, so I asked her to briefly meet with me in the adjoining room to go over them. She sat very still across the table and said only, "He's changing." I waited. Gentle tears rolled down her face. "I miss the strong man I married. He took care of me. It is so hard to see his sadness when I need to start taking over. It's the little things, really. He can't drive or lead me by the arm; I must lead him now. And I know it will only get worse."

Amanda and I talked about her sadness and grief. We discussed support groups, so that she could see that not all people found only sadness in the loss, but sometimes wonder and growth. We arranged to introduce home health aides into the plan of care so that Amanda and Dr. Bob could focus on their relationship and less on activities of daily living. We brought Dr. Bob into the conversation, and he cried with Amanda about the changes they were living through. The family came together to begin rituals to mark transitions and honor the little losses along the way.

---

Anticipatory grief is the process of experiencing bereavement in advance of a loss—usually death. It involves mourning, coping, planning, and restructuring psychologically and socially. It may last for years in families living with dementia as function and cognition decline and caregiving needs increase. Anticipatory grief is reported by family members of individuals newly diagnosed with dementia as well as later in the disease trajectory. Caregivers who live with the individual who has dementia are more likely to experience anticipatory grief. Its onset correlates with greater responsibility for activities that allow a person to remain independent in the community, such as driving, adhering to a medication schedule, and using the phone; frequently occurring dementia-related behaviors, such as sundowning, repeating, or agitation with personal care; and greater lifestyle constraints, such as inability to leave the family member without supervision or to sleep without concerns for safety from wandering.

## The Good and Bad of Anticipatory Grief

Although anticipatory grief is often thought to be negative, some reports suggest that it prepares the caregiver for death and allows for a smoother transition through grief. In one study, depression ratings were highest in family caregivers in the month before the death but returned to significantly lower levels by three months after the death. In contrast, anticipatory grief is reported to account for approximately half of the causes for depression in caregivers and is, therefore, a risk factor for complicated grief. These data suggest another important reason for encouraging interventions for caregiver depression.

## PREPAREDNESS

Family members who are forewarned and prepared for death may be better able to prepare psychologically. Preparedness is not related to the duration or intensity of care that is provided to the individual with a terminal disease; rather, it relates to the family member's perception of death. Twenty-three percent of family members who indicated they felt unprepared for the death of their family member with dementia were two to three times as likely to suffer depression or complicated grief.

## How to Prepare

What does it take to prepare? Is understanding that someone is going to die enough? Some researchers have found the feeling of being unprepared increases when the illness is unpredictable (as is often the case with dementia), when information is inadequate, or when individuals feel insecure in their understanding of the disease. It is important to remember that, to feel prepared, caregivers need information about multiple life concerns. Health care providers may be able to answer some of the medical issues, but other concerns that need to be addressed include psychological issues such as changes in relationships, spiritual issues such as reviewing beliefs on the meaning of death, and practical issues such as funeral or memorial arrangements. Caregivers are encouraged to gather information from a variety of sources, including not just health care providers but also through support groups, reading, and training. Many caregivers report that they didn't ask questions because they were overwhelmed, lost track of what might be important, didn't trust health care providers, or didn't want to be perceived as "ignorant." Armed with this information, it may be useful to keep a running list of questions that can be reviewed at a next visit to see a physician, a social worker, or a spiritual counselor.

## Health Care Providers May Not Initiate the Discussion

In a study of individuals living with advanced dementia who recently entered a nursing home, 90 percent of family members reported being "somewhat or very prepared" for the death of the their family member. In this study, only 15 percent of the health care staff had

had meaningful discussions with family members to assist in preparation, illustrating an area for improvement in the health care community and in the need for families to learn to ask questions. When questions are answered, depression decreases and sense of peace increases. Many health care providers can answer questions or point families to other resources. Be persistent in questioning the entire health care team—physicians, nurses, social workers, and clergy. Your quality of life will benefit.

## RELIEF

### EXPERIENCING SADNESS, GRIEF, AND RELIEF
#### • *Lucinda and Margaret's Story* •

Lucinda was a tall, strong, confident woman. She had come from a family that valued work and owned a thriving family business. Lucinda had taken care of her mother, Margaret, during Margaret's journey with dementia. Margaret's last six months of life had been particularly difficult, with too frequent hospitalizations and delirium, taxing Lucinda's and her sister's strength and resilience. After Margaret died, the family did not hold memorial services for four weeks. After the service, Lucinda described what life over the last several months had been like.

> Mom had been living with dementia so long, I think we all thought she would go on like that forever. Her first bout of pneumonia felt like just a simple blip to us. Your warning that it likely signaled a time of transition toward death fell on deaf ears. We struggled as Mom's behavior and medications were mixed up as she bounced back and forth between the hospital and the rehabilitation center. Finally, we were ready to accept hospice and she died quickly. We were so relieved and actually felt happy that her suffering was over—and that we were out of the hell of the back and forth to the hospital

and rehab. We delayed the memorial so we could recover from being so exhausted and sad. I am glad we did. Now we can properly remember my mom, her life, and our love. She was amazing. So supportive and energetic when we were young and then so brave as she fought to retain her independence as dementia crept into her life. And finally, when she was so fragile—even that allowed my sister and I to grow up, to find ways to help her. I wouldn't change a thing. As sad as it is to lose my mother, I wouldn't change a thing.

Lucinda's family helps us see that relief is a common pattern after periods of long decline or caregiving. Sadness and exhaustion are a part, but the relief, the calm, and the comfort that the family member is no longer struggling or suffering is expected and normal. Many family members who feel guilty that they feel relief are comforted to know that this is typical. In a study of family caregivers' response to death of an individual living with dementia, 90 percent reported that they felt the death was somewhat or very much a relief to the patient and 72 percent felt it was a relief to themselves. Remember that the depression and grief felt immediately after the death usually subside within a month and levels of well-being return to near normal within a year.

## COMPLICATED GRIEF

### NEEDING TO UNDERSTAND AND *ACCEPT DEATH*
#### • *Blake and Poppy's Story* •

Blake was a young version of Poppy. Both were thin, dark skinned, and wide-eyed. Poppy had turned gray and bore wrinkles from a life full of smiles and joy. Before Poppy began to lose his memory, he'd told me stories about Blake. He worried about Blake, his one child "who had failed to launch." He had not understood why

Blake had never really grown up. After some years of roaming the world "aimlessly," Blake had returned to his father's house, unmarried, unemployed, and skittish of life. However, as Poppy's functional status declined, Blake became devoted to Poppy and his care. Blake doted on Poppy's meals, walks, and personal hygiene. Blake was a wonderful, albeit anxious, caregiver. He called the office often to inquire about small rashes, pimples, or sleep changes. Poppy was able to remain home because of the excellent care Blake provided.

As Poppy progressed to the late stages of dementia, I discussed the usual course of death with Blake, but he insisted his father would be fine. But when Blake went to awaken Poppy one morning, he realized Poppy had died in his sleep and had been gone for several hours. Blake spent the day and following night at Poppy's bedside, crying and beseeching Poppy to return. Blake spoke to me a number of times over the next several months, asking me what he had done wrong. No amount of reassurance seemed to resolve Blake's mistaken belief that he had been the cause of Poppy's demise. I spoke to Blake about processing his agony and loss with a therapist, but he refused. I ran into Blake two years later at a hardware store. He reported he was still immobilized by the loss of Poppy, that he couldn't help but dwell daily on how he had let his father down and that he "moved through the day like a zombie, hoping that Poppy would come back to guide him."

---

Complicated grief is defined by the *Diagnostic and Statistical Manual of Mental Disorders (DSM-5)* as a persistent and disruptive yearning or pining for the deceased that impairs important life domains (work, sleep, socialization) and lasts for at least six months. At least four of the eight key symptoms need to be present: (1) trouble accepting the death, (2) inability to trust others since the death, (3) excessive bitterness related to the death, (4) feeling uneasy about moving on, (5) detachment from others who were formerly close, (6) feeling life is meaningless without the deceased, (7) feeling the future holds no prospect for fulfillment without the deceased, and (8) feeling agitated since the death. Aspects of specific complicated grief include retelling the story of the death, having imaginary conversations with the deceased, and avoiding or behaving differently in specific situations (e.g., going to a social event although preferring to remain alone).

## Depression and Anxiety before Death Are Strongest Predictors of Complicated Grief

While most caregivers recover well from the death of a family member, 20 percent of caregivers of those who died from dementia exhibit the symptoms of complicated grief. This may be because depression and anxiety before death are the strongest predictors for complicated grief. Other factors that are also common in caregivers of someone living with dementia include high levels of burden, feeling exhausted, competing responsibilities such as childcare or work, and lack of support. Finally, and somewhat paradoxically, a positive caregiving experience also predicts greater likelihood of complicated grief.

Is anything helpful to avoid complicated grief or treat it once it manifests? Being prepared, as discussed previously, is the best defense against developing complicated grief. If grief is complicated, specific strategies to treat complicated grief are more effective than general treatment of anxiety, depression, or overall grief.

## TRANSITION

---

### FEELING LOST AND LEARNING TO FIND A NEW DIRECTION
#### • Molly's Story •

Molly was a thin woman with a cosmopolitan look. Her mother had died from dementia approximately a year ago, and she wanted to discuss the genetic link of dementia. I had shared in the care of her mother for approximately 10 years. During this time, Molly had been through many changes: a divorce, her children entering adulthood, job changes to provide closer proximity and more flexibility to care for her mother. Molly told me that after her mother passed, she'd been initially tired and took time to rest. Although her energy was restored, she continued to feel the full sadness of losing her mother. "I spent time remembering Mom as a younger mother, the lessons she taught me, what made her laugh, and what made her crazy. Then I marveled at her determination as she lost her memory—she was so stubborn! I love that part of her now. I wish I had seen the positive side then!" We laughed about how Molly usually trailed behind her mother, who led the way, pushing her walker with vigor.

Molly then grew quiet. Once she had grieved her mother's death by celebrating her life, Molly wasn't sure what was next. She had returned to work but found it less interesting. She began taking art classes but did not find them rewarding. She felt no sadness and reported no signs of depression but felt unsure. She knew she wanted something else but, again, wasn't sure what it was. She kept exploring, going to art museums and concerts, sharing adventures with friends to have new experiences, and taking a host of one-day seminars on topics as diverse as meditation to circus performance. Molly said she felt like an investigative reporter, looking for what sparked her interest.

Eventually, she had an opportunity to mentor some high school students and found that she loved interacting with the younger people. She found their ideas stimulating and refreshing and felt her emotionally grounded personality was a valuable counterbalance to their sometimes misguided enthusiasm. Molly glowed as she reported working with the high school counselor to find ways to stay involved, and she'd already started taking courses and internships to obtain certification in social work and counseling. It was a joy to see Molly's light as she described her transformation and new direction for the next phase of her life.

## Transitions Are the Psychological Process of Change

William Bridges, a leading author and expert in change and transition, describes *change* as a situation, such as a shift in job responsibilities or death of a spouse, and *transition* as the psychological process of incorporating the change into your personal outlook and worldview. Transition occurs either leading up to a change or as a reaction to it. Bridges says we go through an inner reorientation and self-redefinition to incorporate changes into our lives. He posits that, in the United States, we have sped life up and lost faith that change will lead to something good. The American resistance and uneasiness with change comes from the distressing feeling that upheaval is fraught with unknown outcome. Older and other societies have prepared effectively for change with rituals, for example, seasonal rituals about birth and death or spiritual rituals at the time of entering adulthood.

Bridges's theory of personal development views transition as a natural process of growth, with numerous turning points on its path. He highlights that growth is not linear but involves many starts and stops along the way that ultimately lead to acceptance and action. He describes a three-phase process to the psychological changes of transition: endings, neutral zone, and new beginnings.

## Endings Lead to New Beginnings, with an Incubation Gap In-Between

Endings are often skirted because they may be painful. Death can be a particularly painful ending. But we see that, for most people, a time of bereavement is brief and bittersweet, resulting in beautiful and heartfelt memories, along with small rituals to keep the lost in our hearts and daily lives in a new way. We intuitively realize that letting go of the old patterns that involved the deceased is necessary to move forward. Some do this easily and quickly, while others require a more measured and gradual letting go. Bridges recommends touring the losses in your life (for example, loss of something physical, relationships, jobs, hobbies) and how you have dealt with them along the way. This review may help you identify how you respond to losses, which can help you undergo change and transitions. It may also help you remember that endings lead to new beginnings, either expected or unexpected. Realizing that endings open you to a new beginning often eases the way to letting go and personal growth.

When the change involves the end of a relationship, as it does with the death of a family member, Bridges recommends several steps to assist in this transition. Allow yourself time for the inner change that will be required at the end of your family member's life. While you work through this change, perhaps you can arrange for a few temporary ways to ease your other responsibilities, such as delegating some decisions to others or delaying some decisions for a time. Be sure not to act hastily in this time of transition. Respect that times of change require some contemplation before making a large shift. Pampering yourself in small ways can also ease the transition. I found that taking time to just sit and drink tea helped to find calmness. This pampering fills one of Bridges's other recommendations, which is to take a time-out. Use this time to look for the silver lining in the change you didn't ask for.

The next phase of transition is what Bridges calls the neutral zone, or in-between the ending and the new beginning. Several cultures separate the individual going through the transition from the community during this phase. For example, an individual might go into the forest or desert to fast, to see visions, to have time to dream (literally and figuratively), or to shed the old ways and prepare for new ones.

In American culture, we have not ritualized the neutral zone, but it is not uncommon for people to take a long vacation, to go on a retreat, or to find a way to "get away from it all." In this time of in-between, unusual happenings may be encountered and, when listened to, may be a source of guidance. In Joan Didion's memoir, *The Year of Magical Thinking*, she describes vivid dreams, guidance, and discussions with her husband in the year after his death. I spoke with many friends and patients after reading this book and nearly all described events that they interpreted as symbolic, odd, and "too real to be a coincidence," which they found comforting and calming. Dan Siegel, PhD, a neuroscientist, asks his seminar audiences about experiences with "others, alive or dead, in which you know there is a connection and knowing that occurred without being physically present together." Half the crowd (of hundreds) always raise their hands. My grieving patients find it comforting when I admit to them that I too have had "other worldly experiences" (sensing and smelling my father's cologne at an anxious time while performing a medical procedure; hearing my mother's voice during meditation; finding a note from my mother tucked into a book supporting me and telling me to "hang in there"— a note I had never seen before) and use them as guidance and comfort. My spiritual colleagues concur that time for contemplation has been used by individuals, mystics, clergy, and peasants for thousands of years.

Bridges also describes activities that can assist in the neutral zone. He recommends accepting the need for a time in the neutral zone, finding a regular time and place to be alone, taking time to journal about your experiences in the neutral zone (to gain perspective), and reviewing where your life has been and where you would like it to go. This is a time for inner exploration and germination for the new beginning that is coming.

### New Interests or Transformations May Seem to Come on Quickly after Incubation

The final stage of a transition is the new beginning. Bridges ponders how we know when we've completely made an end to something and spent adequate time in the neutral zone. Using analogies to plantings can help us understand this process. When the ground has been made ready, the seeds are in place, and there has been an adequate amount of sun and rain, new beginnings happen. There is no sign or specific time frame that makes it right. The time is probably right when ideas or situations are interesting. Remember the story of Molly and how she tried many different activities. With these new experiences, a few "stuck" and allowed Molly to imagine and begin a new, renewed life. When my mother entered her later years of dementia, it was the first time in my 25-year career in medicine that I slowed down the pace. I only then became aware that I had allowed certain aspects of my life to fall out of balance. When my mother's life ended, I knew it was time to realign my life as well. If not for the time I spent sitting and saying goodbye to her and opening myself to other family members, friends, and caregivers during this time, I would not have had the opportunity for renewal.

## NEW BEGINNINGS

It is now several years since the death of my mother, and I can say that her final years and death were one of the most meaningful gifts she gave me. I was opened to new transitions. Much like Molly, I entered a time when I acknowledged endings, entered a period in the neutral zone of uncertainty and exploration, and emerged into new beginnings in both my work and personal life. By taking the time to dwell in the neutral zone, I made psychological shifts that allowed healing and growth. I've entered a life that I live much more fully, better balancing the needs of mind, body, and spirit. The process truly broke my heart open from a place of fear and worry. My hope is that the journey with dementia, in all its ups and downs, can be as fulfilling for you as it was for me and my family.

---

### POINTS TO REMEMBER

---

▸ Most individuals handle grief with resilience. Initial sadness is interspersed with laughter and fond memories, leading to acceptance and finally living well.

▸ Caregivers can approach grief well by using several strategies. These include anticipating and partially grieving before the death, being prepared and understanding that the death is imminent and necessary, and feeling relief that the deceased is no longer suffering and that the burden of caregiving has come to a close.

▶ Complicated grief occurs in 20–30 percent of caregivers of those who died with advanced dementia. The strongest predictor of complicated grief is depression in the caregiver.

▶ Specific treatment strategies to address complicated grief are more successful than general treatments for depression.

▶ It is common to enter a time of transition after the loss of an important relationship, especially when caregiving was involved.

▶ Times of loss and endings often open our lives to personal growth and transformation.

---

### ACTION PLAN

▶ Realize that grief is aided by preparation. Take time to journal about the impending death of your family member and your thoughts on the necessity and positive attributes of death.

▶ Take time for transition after the death of your family member: the ending, the neutral zone, and a new beginning. Take time to rest and explore new interests before embarking in a new direction. Journal your dreams and new interests.

---

### ADDITIONAL READING AND RESOURCES

▶ *The Other Side of Sadness: What the New Science of Bereavement Tells Us about Life after Loss*, by George A. Bonanno

This book outlines clearly what is known about bereavement, the typical resilient recovery, and when this may not occur. Although this book does not focus on dementia, it does have discussions that focus on grief in those who have served as a caregiver.

▶ *Transitions: Making Sense of Life's Changes*, by William Bridges

This classic describes the underlying and universal pattern of transition: endings, neutral zone, and new beginnings. The beautifully written book uses the classic literature and mythology to assist in understanding the patterns of change.

# Index